NOTES IN NEUROANAESTHESIA
AND CRITICAL CARE

Dedication

To our families whose understanding, patience and support has made this book possible.

NOTES IN NEUROANAESTHESIA AND CRITICAL CARE

Edited by

Arun K. Gupta MBBS MA FRCA
Director of Neuro-critical care and Consultant in Anaesthesia
Associate Lecturer
Addenbrooke's Hospital
Cambridge

Andrew C. Summors BSc (HONS) MBBS (HONS) FRCA
Formerly Specialist Registrar and Fellow in Neuroanaesthesia
Addenbrooke's Hospital
Cambridge
Consultant in Anaesthesia and Critical Care
Nevill Hall Hospital
Abergavenny
Wales

GMM

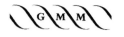

© 2001

GREENWICH MEDICAL MEDIA LTD
137 Euston Road
London
NW1 2AA

ISBN 1 84110 035 8

First published 2001

Distributed worldwide by
Plymbridge Distributors Ltd

Typeset by Phoenix Photosetting, Chatham, Kent
Printed by Ashford Colour Press Ltd, Hants

Contents

Anatomy

Physiology

Pharmacology

Neuroanaesthesia

Neurointensive care

Monitoring

Contributors

Rowan Burnstein
FRCA
Specialist Registrar
University of Cambridge

Ian Calder
DRCOG FRCA
Consultant Anaesthetist
The National Hospital for Neurology and
Neurosurgery, and The Royal Free Hospital
Queen Square, London

Alisdair Coles
BA BM BCh MRCP PhD
Wellcome Advanced Fellow, Neurology
Cambridge University

Jonathan Coles
FRCA
Addenbrooke's Hospital,
Cambridge

Marek Czosnyka
PhD
Snr Research Scientist
University of Cambridge

Patrick Doyle
Specialist Registrar
FRCA
Addenbrooke's Hospital,
Cambridge

Cathy Duffy
FRCA
Consultant Anaesthetist
Addenbrooke's Hospital,
Cambridge

Richard Erskine
FRCA
Consultant Anaesthetist
Addenbrooke's Hospital,
Cambridge

Jonathan H. Gillard
BSc, MD FRCR
Clinical Lecturer
Univ Dept of Radiology
Addenbrooke's Hospital,
Cambridge

Craig Goldsack
BSc MRCP FRCA
Consultant Anaesthetist
University College London Hospitals
London

Ken Grixti
FRCA
Specialist Registrar
Addenbrooke's Hospital,
Cambridge

Arun K. Gupta
MA FRCA
Director of Neuro-critical care
Associate Lecturer
University of Cambridge
Addenbrooke's Hospital,
Cambridge

Sanjeeva Gupta
FRCA
Consultant in Chronic Pain
Bradford Hospital,
Yorkshire

Nicholas P. Hirsch
FRCA
Consultant Neuroanaesthetist
Harris Neurorespiratory Intensive Care Unit
The National Hospital for Neurology and
Neurosurgery,
Queen Square, London

P. J. A. Hutchinson
FRCS
Specialist Registrar
Addenbrooke's Hospital,
Cambridge

Rodney Laing
MA MD FRCS (SN)
Consultant Neurosurgeon
Addenbrooke's Hospital,
Cambridge

Tim Leary
FRCA
Specialist Registrar
Addenbrooke's Hospital, Cambridge

Brian McNamara
MRCP
Specialist Registrar
Addenbrooke's Hospital,
Cambridge

Basil Matta
FRCA
Director of Perioperative Services
Addenbrooke's Hospital,
Cambridge

David K. Menon
MD PhD FRCP FRCA F Med Sci
Professor of Anaesthesia
University of Cambridge

Quentin J. W. Milner
FRCA
Consultant Anaesthetist
Portsmouth Hospitals,
Hants

Joseph Monteiro
MD
Consultant Anesthesiologist
Hinduja National Hospital and
Medical Research Centre,
Bombay, India

Ivan Ng
FRCS
Co-Director of Neurosciences ICU
National Neuroscience Institute
Singapore

Phil Popham
MD FRCA
Chairman
Dept of Anaesthesia
Addenbrooke's Hospital,
Cambridge

Mahesh Prabhu
FRCA
Specialist Registrar
Addenbrooke's Hospital,
Cambridge

Sandra Rees-Pedlar
BSc (Hons) PG Cert
Sister, Neurointensive Care
Addenbrooke's Hospital,
Cambridge

Siva Senthuran
FRCA
Specialist Registrar
Addenbrooke's Hospital,
Cambridge

Ravi Shankar
Specialist Registrar
Addenbrooke's Hospital,
Cambridge

Jay Shapiro
MD
Associate Professor
Director of Pediatric Anaesthesia
Medical College of Virginia,
Richmond, VA
USA

Martin Smith
FRCA
Consultant Neuroanaesthetist and Honorary
Lecturer in Anaesthesia
The National Hospital for Neurology and
Neurosurgery,
University College London Hospitals
Queen Square, London

Andrew C. Summors
BSc FRCA
Formerly Specialist Registrar and Fellow in
Neuroanaesthesia
Addenbrooke's Hospital,
Cambridge

Consultant in Anaesthesia and Critical Care
Nevill Hall Hospital
Abergavenny
Wales

Atul Swami
MRCP FRCA
Consultant Anaesthetist
Addenbrooke's Hospital,
Cambridge

John M. Turner
MA FRCA
Consultant in Anaesthesia and Neurointensive Care
Addenbrooke's Hospital,
Cambridge

John Ulatowski
MD PhD MBA
Vice Chairman, Clinical Affairs
Associate Professor, Anesthesiology/
Critical Care Medicine
Johns Hopkins Medical Institutions,
Baltimore, MD
USA

Sally Walters
BSc
Senior Sister
Neurointensive Care
Addenbrooke's Hospital,
Cambridge

Charles Williams
MD
Assistant Professor
Director of Neuroanesthesiology
Medical College of Virginia,
Richmond, VA
USA

Preface

Anaesthetists in training are expected to acquire an extensive knowledge of a number of diverse specialities in a short period of time. During their period of training in neuroanaesthesia and neuro-critical care, they are expected to remind themselves of many basic principles including neuroanatomy, neurophysiology and pharmacology. In addition they need to understand new concepts to a sufficient depth to be able to apply them in the clinical setting.

In our experience, few trainees will contemplate reading a detailed textbook and we are frequently asked to recommend a more appropriate text on the subject. We therefore decided to collate short notes on specific topics in neuroanaesthesia and critical care for use by anaesthetists working toward their professional examinations and to stimulate discussion and teaching between trainees and faculty. This book is a compilation of these short notes.

The book is not intended to be a complete reference text, of which there are many, but primarily to provide essential information and key references so that further detailed information can be found if required. In this way we hope that that the book will be a useful practical guide to clinical practice.

Although this book is aimed at trainee anaesthetists preparing for their final FRCA exam, it may be of value as a revision aid for all practising anaesthetists, medical and nursing staff in Intensive Care Units, junior doctors in neurology and neurosurgery as well as medical students. Staff in non-neurosurgical centres who manage neurologically injured patients in their units or who have to transfer patients to other units will also find this book valuable.

Contributors have come from both trainee and faculty grades in an attempt to convey the essential information as succinctly as possible. The key points at the end of each chapter should help as a quick 'aide memoire'.

A. K. G.
A. S.
February 2001

Acknowledgements

We are indebted to all our colleagues who have contributed their knowledge and expertise in preparing this book, in particular Philip Ball, Senior Medical Artist at Addenbrooke's Hospital for his skill in preparing many of the illustrations. We are also grateful to the authors, publishers and editors for permission to reproduce or modify various tables and figures used.

Cover image courtesy of Philips Medical Systems

Abbreviations

ACA	anterior cerebral artery		EEG	electroencephalogram
ACh	acetylcholine		EMG	electromyogram
AChR	acetylcholine receptor		ETT	endotracheal tube
ACTH	adrenocorticotropic hormone		GBS	Guillain–Barré syndrome
ADH	antidiuretic hormone		GCS	Glasgow coma scale
AJDO$_2$	arterio-jugular differences in O$_2$ content		GCSC	generalised convulsive status epilepticus
ANF	atrial natriuretic factor		GTN	glyceral trinitrate
AVM	arteriovenous malformation		GH	growth hormone
BAEP	brainstem auditory evoked potential		Hb	haemoglobin
			HbO$_2$	oxygenated Hb
BBB	blood–brain barrier		HI	head injury
BP	blood pressure		ICA	internal carotid artery
BSR	burst suppression ratio		ICH	intracranial haemorrhage
CBF	cerebral blood flow		ICP	intracranial pressure
CBV	cerebral blood volume		IHD	ischaemic heart disease
CEA	carotid endarterectomy		IJV	internal jugular vein
CFM	cerebral function monitoring		LDF	laser Doppler flowmetry
CMAP	compound motor action potential		MAP	mean arterial pressure
CMR/CMRO$_2$	cerebral metabolic rate of oxygen		MABP	mean arterial blood pressure
CN	cranial nerve		MCA	middle cerebral artery
CNS	central nervous system		MCAFvx	middle cerebral artery flow velocity
CPP	cerebral perfusion pressure		MMC	myelomeningocele
CSF	cerebrospinal fluid		MRI	magnetic resonance imaging
CT	computed tomography		MRS	magnetic resonance spectroscopy
CTG	cardiotocography		NIRS	near infrared spectroscopy
CVP	central venous pressure		NO	nitric oxide
CVR	cerebrovascular resistance		N$_2$O	nitrous oxide
DAI	diffuse axonal injury		PaO$_2$	arterial oxygen tension
DI	diabetes insipidus		PaCO$_2$	arterial carbon dioxide tension
DIC	disseminated intravascular coagulation		PbO$_2$	brain tissue oxygen tension
			PCA	posterior cerebral artery
ECA	external carotid artery		PCoA	posterior communicating artery
ECG	electrocardiogram		PEG	percutaneous gastrostomy
ECoG	electrocorticogram		PEEP	positive end-expiratory pressure
EDH	extradural haematoma		PICA	posterior-inferior cerebellar artery

rCBF	regional cerebral blood flow	SjvO$_2$	jugular bulb oxygen saturation
RIND	reversible ischaemic neurologic deficits	SNP	sodium nitroprusside
		SPECT	single photon emission computed tomography
rtPA	recombinant tissue plasminogen activator	SSEP	somatosensory evoked potential
SAH	subarachnoid haemorrhage	TCD	transcranial Doppler
SAP	sensory action potential		ultrasonography
SCI	spinal cord injury	TIA	transient ischaemic attack
SCPP	spinal cord perfusion pressure	TSH	thyroid-stimulating hormone
SDH	subdural haematoma	VP	venous pressure
SEP	somatosensory evoked potential	V-P	ventriculo-peritoneal
SIADH	syndrome of inappropriate antidiuretic hormone secretion	VEP	visual evoked potential
		WBC	white blood cell

Section 1

ANATOMY

1

ANATOMY OF THE BRAIN AND SPINAL CORD

C. Williams

GENERAL ORGANISATION

The central nervous system (CNS) can be divided into brainstem, cerebellum, cerebrum and spinal cord.

A fibrous membrane surrounds the entire CNS and its cerebrospinal fluid (CSF), and is composed of three layers, collectively known as the meninges. The outermost layer is the dura, which adheres to the inner surface of the skull and continues down to the tip of the spinal cord (filum terminale). While neural tissue itself does not generally sense pain, the dura does, and the sympathetic discharge from dural incision can lead to unwanted rises in blood pressure and heart rate if not anticipated. The innermost layer is the pia, which is in contact with the neural tissues of the CNS. The middle layer is called the arachnoid, and the trabeculated space between the arachnoid and pia membranes contains CSF. Blood vessels on the outside of the dura service the meninges itself, and disruption of these vessels causes epidural hematomas. The pia supports blood vessels that service the metabolically active neural tissues, and disruption of these vessels cause subdural hematomas. Around the base of the brain, these subdural (pial) vessels form a network called the Circle of Willis that, in most patients, assures a collateral supply of blood (see Chapter 2 for blood supply to the brain).

ANATOMY OF THE BRAINSTEM (FIG. 1.1)

The brainstem is a small but extremely important structure, and has primarily three functions.

Firstly, it is a conduit for transmitting signals back and forth from the cerebrum and cerebellum to the spinal cord, e.g. the long motor fibres (corticospinal tracts) run along the anterior aspect of the brainstem in the cerebral peduncles, cross the midline in the pyramids, and enter the top of the spinal cord. Sensory pathways pursue similar courses, although most do not cross the midline here. Secondly, the 12 cranial nerves (CN) and their nuclei are found in the brainstem. These nerves control the motor and sensory functions of the head, face and most of the neck Table 1.1. The vagus nerve (CN X) also communicates with the chest, heart and abdomen, and if compressed in the carotid sheath during carotid endarterectomy or anterior cervical fusion, can cause bradycardia. Since these nerves and nuclei are so closely located in and around the brainstem, problems in this area rarely affect only one cranial nerve. Compression of the facial nerve (CN VII) by an acoustic neuroma (on CN VIII) is common, so during surgical resection of this tumour, both facial electromyogram (EMG) and evoked brainstem auditory monitoring may be required. Even simple manipulation of the trigeminal nerve (CN V) easily affects the nearby nucleus ambiguus (of CN X), causing bradycardia. Lastly, management of the essential involuntary functions of heart rate, blood pressure and respiratory rate occurs in the reticular networks of the brainstem, with input from the hypothalamus. Considering the overall importance of

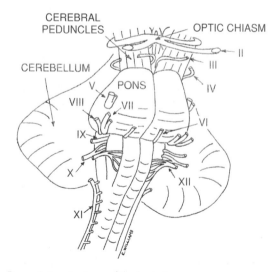

Figure 1.1   Anatomy of the brainstem

Table 1.1 The cranial nerves and their functions		
	Cranial Nerve	Function
I	Olfactory	Smell
II	Optic	Vision
III	Oculomotor	Moves eyes, constricts pupils, opens eyelids
IV	Trochlear	Moves eyes
V	Trigeminal	Sensory to face, chews
VI	Abducens	Moves eyes
VII	Facial	Motor to face, taste, closes eyelids
VIII	Vestibulocochlear	Hears, regulates balance
IX	Glossopharyngeal	Swallows, sensory to posterior pharynx, controls salivation
X	Vagus	Sensory to airway and abdominal viscera, parasympathetic to heart
XI	Accessory	Lifts shoulders, rotates head
XII	Hypoglossal	Motor to tongue

brainstem function, it is easy to see why strokes or injury to the brainstem have such devastating effects to the patient.

ANATOMY OF THE CEREBELLUM AND DEEP STRUCTURES OF THE BRAIN

Sitting atop the brainstem are the deep brain structures of the hypothalamus, thalamus and basal ganglia. These are primarily relay and control stations for the autonomic and endocrine nervous systems and receive enormous amounts of sensory input. Pathology here is seldom surgically correctable, with the notable exceptions of thalamotomies for tremors (usually Parkinsonian), or pituitary surgery.

The cerebellum, which lies posterior to the brainstem, functions primarily in the regulation of fine motor control. Dysfunction is generally characterised by awkwardness of intentional movements or tremors. Together with the brainstem it sits at the bottom of the skull in the posterior fossa and is covered by a dural sheet (the tentorum) that separates it from the cerebrum. Compared to the cerebral vault, the posterior fossa is small, and a small increase in volume here can quickly compress the brainstem. Postoperative blood pressure elevation may lead to haematoma following surgery in this area.

ANATOMY OF THE CEREBRUM (FIG. 1.2)

The hemispheres of the cerebrum can each be divided into four major areas called lobes. The frontal lobes lie over the orbital bones and are responsible for abstract thinking, voluntary eye movements, mature judgements and self-control. They are separated from the more posterior parietal lobes by a vertical groove called the central sulcus, and the strip of frontal cortex running just anterior to the sulcus is the primary motor control centre. Control of the contralateral lower extremity is more rostral on this strip (supplied by the anterior cerebral artery), and control of the contralateral upper extremity and face is more caudal (supplied by the middle cerebral artery). The primary sensory cortex exists in a similar arrangement on the strip of parietal cortex just posterior to the sulcus, and is responsible for discerning fine touch, determining proprioception, and for recognising the source, quality and severity of pain and temperature. The area around the most posterior tip of the brain (occipital lobe) is the visual cortex and is used for the interpretation of sight and for high-level control of the occulomotor complex. Extending forward and laterally is the temporal lobe, whose deeper structures form the limbic systems that play important roles in memory and learning.

Although the cerebrum is bilaterally symmetrical in appearance, its function is not. Almost all right-handed people are left-brain dominant, but only 60–70% of left-handed people are right-brain dominant. Dominance can be determined by a WADA test (selectively anaesthetising each temporal lobe), and can be especially important for temporal lobe resections since language interpretation (Wernicke's area) and motor speech centres (Broca's area) are found primarily in the fronto-temporal regions of the dominant hemisphere.

ANATOMY OF THE SPINAL CORD (FIG. 1.3)

Although there are many identifiable ascending and descending neuronal tracts in the spinal cord, only three hold major clinical significance.

The only important *descending* tract is the corticospinal tract, which runs from the brain's motor cortex (precentral gyrus), through the internal capsule and cerebral peduncles, across to the contralateral side via the pyramidal decussation, and down the lateral columns of the spinal cord. Motor nerve roots come off of the spinal cord periodically and are bundled together as peripheral nerves that pass through each spinal foramina as they continue on to the body's muscles. Although there are 30 vertebral bones, there are actually 31 pairs of spinal nerves. Since the top seven cervical nerves exit over their corresponding seven vertebrae, and all of the nerves below the top-most thoracic level exit under their corresponding vertebrae, an extra cervical nerve (C8) exists between the C7 and T1 vertebrae.

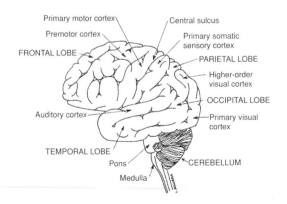

Figure 1.2   Gross anatomy of the cerebrum

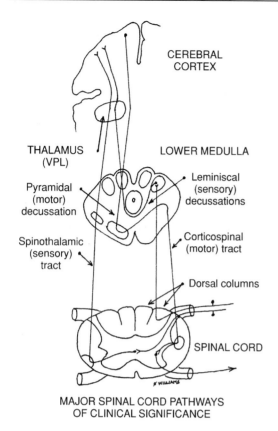

CEREBRAL
CORTEX

THALAMUS
(VPL)

LOWER MEDULLA

Pyramidal
(motor)
decussation

Leminiscal
(sensory)
decussations

Spinothalamic
(sensory)
tract

Corticospinal
(motor) tract

Dorsal columns

SPINAL CORD

Ø WILLIAMS

MAJOR SPINAL CORD PATHWAYS
OF CLINICAL SIGNIFICANCE

Figure 1.3   Major spinal cord pathways of clinical significance

For any given muscle target, this entire pathway comprises only two cells: the upper motor neurone runs from the brain to the appropriate spinal cord level, and the lower motor neurone runs from the spinal cord to the muscle. Injury or disease affecting the lower motor neurone results in a focal weakness, fasciculation, wasting and hyporeflexia, while pathology affecting the upper motor neurones of the spinothalamic tract produces spasticity and hyper-reflexia to all muscles serviced by neurones below the level of injury. It is however, clinically difficult to correlate spinal cord levels with specific motor innervation of the trunk, so sensory losses may be a more valuable localising tool when the lesion is above the first lumbar level.

The *first* of the two major *ascending* neuronal tracts is the lateral spinothalamic tract. Information about pain, temperature and crude touch from peripheral nerves enters the posterior horn of the spinal cord, crosses to the contralateral side of the cord one or two levels above where it entered, and is sent rostrally to the brain's sensory cortex (postcentral gyrus) after passing through the thalamus. While in the thoracic and cervical spinal cord, the lateral spinothalamic tract maintains a somatotopic organisation, as nerve fibres originating in the lowermost levels are pushed laterally by fibres entering from successively higher levels. This organisation allows neurosurgeons to sometimes perform very selective cordotomies to treat intractable pelvic or leg pain, and to help localise lateral spinal cord lesions. Furthermore, expanding central cord lesions will compress the medial fibres from higher levels first, often sparing the more lateral fibres from the sacrum.

The *second* of the two major *ascending* neuronal tracts, the dorsal column-medial leminiscal system, carries information about two-point discrimination, joint position and vibration up the ipsilateral dorsal columns to a contralateral crossover point in the medulla. From there, the signal is relayed through the thalamus to the brain's primary sensory cortex (post-central gyrus).

The anterior and central portions of the spinal cord (including the corticospinal and lateral spinothalamic tracts) are supplied with blood from the anterior spinal artery, which arises from the vertebral arteries at the base of the brain rostrally and the arteria magna of Adamkewicz (a low-thoracic branch of the aorta) caudally. Paired, poorly defined posterior spinal arteries, however, service the dorsal columns. This arrangement can lead to differential ischaemia of the spinal cord, if only one of the arterial systems is disrupted. Anterior cord syndromes, for example, are seen in cervical spine hyperflexion injuries, displaced spinal fractures, posteriorly herniated disks or ischaemia from anterior spinal artery occlusion. It produces injury to the lateral spinothalamic and corticospinal tracts while sparing the dorsal columns and typically causes immediate paralysis with loss of pain and temperature sensation below the level of the lesion; light touch and vibration and joint position senses are preserved throughout. Radicular branches from the posterior spinal arteries (arising from the posterior inferior cerebellar arteries or the vertebral arteries) service the posterior one-third of the spinal cord. As they are so much more widely anastamosed than their anterior counterparts, injury to any one of them will not necessarily result in cord ischaemia. Spinal cord blood flow is autoregulated in similar fashion to cerebral blood flow.

Complete and incomplete sectioning of the spinal cord produces characteristic clinical pictures based upon the extent of damage done to these three major neuronal tracts. Traumatic complete sectioning of the cord produces immediate loss of voluntary movement and sensation below the level of the injury followed by distal hyperreflexia and muscular spasticity after several weeks. A hemisection of the cord produces the *Brown–Séquard syndrome*, which has four parts:

1. Corticospinal tract injury produces ipsilateral motor loss below the lesion.
2. Dorsal column injury produces ipsilateral sensory loss to joint position, two-point discrimination, and vibration below the lesion.
3. Lateral spinothalamic tract injury produces contralateral loss of pain, temperature and crude touch below a point one to two levels above the lesion.

4. The sympathetic system is commonly also damaged in high hemisections, producing an ipsilateral Horner's syndrome (miosis and ptosis).

FURTHER READING

Goldberg S. Clinical neuroanatomy made ridiculously simple. Miami, Florida: MedMaster, 1997

Pansky B, Allen DJ. Review of neuroscience. New York: Macmillan, 1980

Rowland LP. Clinical syndromes of the spinal cord and brain stem. In: Kandel ER, Schwartz JH, Jessell TM (eds) Principles of neural science, 3rd Edn. Norwalk, Connecticut: Appleton & Lange, 1991, pp. 711–720

2

CEREBRAL CIRCULATION

R. Burnstein

INTRODUCTION

The brain has the highest metabolic requirements of any organ in the body. It receives 14% of the resting cardiac output in the adult (approximately 700 ml/min) and accounts for 20% of basal oxygen consumption (about 50 ml/min). Blood flow within the brain is variable with flow in the grey matter (110 ml/100 g tissue/min) on average 5 times that in white matter (22 ml/100 g/min).

ARTERIAL BLOOD SUPPLY

The arterial supply to the brain is from both right and left internal carotid arteries (ICAs) supplying the anterior two-thirds of the cerebral hemispheres and the vertebrobasilar system, which supplies the brainstem and the posterior regions of the hemispheres.

The *common carotid artery* lies in the neck within the carotid sheath medial to the *internal jugular vein* (IJV) with the *vagus nerve* posteriorly between them. The sympathetic trunk runs behind the artery but outside the sheath. At approximately the level of the thyroid cartilage the common carotid artery bifurcates into ICA and *external carotid artery* (ECA).

Just above the bifurcation, the ECA passes between the ICA and the pharyngeal wall. It supplies the soft tissues of the neck, eye, face and scalp. The ICA continues to pass vertically upwards in the neck within the carotid sheath giving off no branches. It is superficial at first in the carotid triangle, but then passes deeper, medial to the posterior belly of the digastric muscle. At its origin is a fusiform dilatation known as the carotid sinus. The walls of the sinus contain baroreceptors that are stimulated by changes in blood pressure. The ICA enters the skull through the foramen lacerum and turns anteriorly through the cavernous sinus in the carotid groove on the side of the sphenoid body.

Each ICA gives rise to a *posterior communicating artery* (PCoA) before ending by dividing into the *anterior cerebral artery* (ACA) and *middle cerebral artery* (MCA). The ACA runs medially then superiorly, supplying the undersurface of the frontal lobe and the medial neostriatum. The MCA turns laterally from its origin, immediately giving rise to a series of small penetrating branches, the *lenticulostriate arteries*. These arteries are the only supply to the lateral part of the striatum. The MCA continues to run laterally where it divides into several major branches carrying blood to the lateral surfaces of the frontal, temporal and parietal lobes.

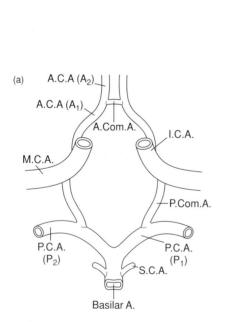

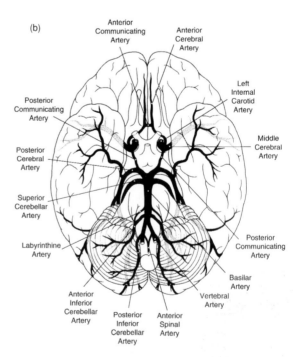

Figure 2.1a & b   (a) Anatomy of the Circle of Willis. The classic polygonal ring is found in less than 50% of brains. ICA, internal carotid artery, ACA, anterior cerebral artery, MCA, middle cerebral artery, PCA, posterior cerebral artery, ACoA, anterior communicating artery, PCoA, posterior communicating artery, SCA, superior cerebellar artery. (b) Relationship of Circle of Willis and branches to the base of the brain

The *vertebral arteries* arise from the *subclavian arteries* at the base of the neck. They fuse to form the *basilar artery* at the level of the pontomedullary junction. The basilar artery lies on the ventral surface of the brainstem and supplies blood to the pons, midbrain and cerebellum. At the level of the midbrain the artery bifurcates to form two large *posterior cerebral arteries* (PCAs), from which several small branches arise including the small PCoAs.

The anastomoses between the internal carotid system and the vertebrobasilar systems form the *Circle of Willis* (Fig. 2.1). It is located in the interpenduncular cistern and encloses the optic chiasm, pituitary stalk and mamillary bodies. The 'classic' polygonal anastomotic ring (Fig. 2.1a), however, is found in less than 50% of brains. The vessels of the Circle send branches supplying superficial tissue as well as long penetrating branches supplying deep grey matter structures. These deep penetrating branches are functional end arteries and although there are anastomoses between distal branches of cerebral and cerebellar arteries, the concept of boundary zone (i.e. watershed) ischaemia is important. Global cerebral ischaemia with systemic hypotension (e.g. cardiac arrest), typically produces lesions in areas where the zones of blood supply from two vessels meet – between the cortical areas of distribution of the ACA, MCA and PCA and between the superior cerebellar and posterior inferior cerebellar arteries. However, the presence of anatomical variations may substantially modify patterns of infarction following large vessel occlusion. Figure 2.2 demonstrates the areas supplied by the cerebral arteries.

The majority of intracranial aneurysms may be found in the following sites:

- Anterior communicating (25%);
- Internal carotid (22%);
- Middle cerebral (25%);
- Internal carotid bifurcation (4%);
- Basilar bifurcation (7%).

VENOUS DRAINAGE

Venous drainage (Fig. 2.3) comprises a series of external and internal veins, which drain into the *venous sinuses*. The venous sinuses are endothelialised channels, continuous with the endothelial surface of the veins, but which lie between folds of dura mater. They have no valves and their walls are devoid of muscular tissue. The sinuses drain into the internal jugular vein (IJV), which are continuous with the *sigmoid sinus* at the jugular foramen. The IJV has a 'bulb' at its upper end, which is an enlargement in the wall of the vein. At the level of the *jugular bulb* the IJVs receive minimal venous return from extracranial tissue and measurement of oxygen saturation ($SjvO_2$) at this level can be used as a measure of cerebral oxygenation. Current evidence suggests that about 70% of the flow to each vein are from ipsilateral tissue, 3% from extracranial tissue and the remainder from the contralateral hemisphere.

Many clinicians are concerned that internal jugular central lines will impair venous drainage from the

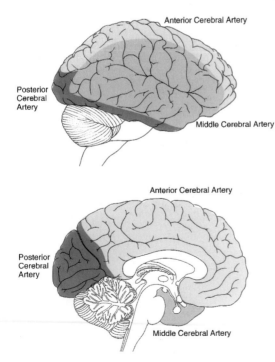

Figure 2.2   Areas supplied by the cerebral arteries

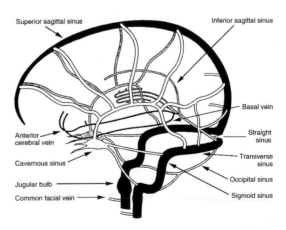

Figure 2.3   Venous drainage of the brain

brain and that this impairment may lead to increased bleeding into the surgical site or increased intracranial pressure in the intact skull of a susceptible patient. The evidence to support this as being clinically relevant is weak.

MICROCIRCULATION

The architecture of the cerebral microvasculature is highly organised. Pial vessels on the surface of the brain give rise to arterioles that penetrate the brain at right angles. These give rise to capillaries at all laminar levels. Each arteriole supplies a hexagonal column of tissue with overlapping boundary zones resulting in columnar patterns of local blood flow. This parallels the columnar arrangement seen within neuronal groups and physiological functional units. Capillary density in the adult is related to the number of synapses and can be closely correlated with the regional level of oxidative metabolism.

BLOOD–BRAIN BARRIER

Endothelial cells in cerebral capillaries contain specialised tight junctions. As a result the cerebral capillary endothelium has a high electrical resistance and is relatively impermeable. Passage of substances across the intact blood–brain barrier (BBB) is predominantly a function of lipid solubility and the presence of active transport systems.

The BBB maintains tight control of ionic distribution in the extracellular fluid of the brain. Four areas, the circumventricular organs, which include the posterior pituitary gland, lie outside the blood–brain barrier.

KEY POINTS

- The brain has the highest metabolic requirement of any organ.
- The arterial supply is from the carotid arteries and the vertebrobasilar system.
- The arteries anatomose in the Circle of Willis.
- Venous drainage occurs through epithelialised venous sinuses draining into the internal jugular veins.
- The microcirculation is highly organised with capillary density correlated with functional activity.
- The blood–brain barrier is maintained by the capillary endothelium and is highly impermeable.

FURTHER READING

Williams PL (ed). Gray's Anatomy, 38th Edn. Edinburgh: Churchill Livingstone, 1995

Menon DK. Cerebral circulation. In: Cardiovascular physiology. London: BMJ Publishing Group, 1999

3

ANATOMY OF THE POSTERIOR FOSSA

A. Swami

INTRODUCTION

The posterior cranial fossa is almost circular in outline and is the largest and deepest of the three cranial fossae (Fig. 3.1) (the others being anterior and middle fossae). It contains the cerebellum and brainstem, which are covered by a dural sheet (the tentorium cerebelli) which separates it from the cerebrum.

The **boundaries** of the posterior fossa are as follows:

- **Anteriorly** lies the dorsum sellae, the clivus, the posterior part of sphenoid and the basilar part of the occipital bone.
- **Posteriorly** lies the squamous part of the occipital bone, the transverse sinus and the superior sagittal sinus.
- **Laterally** lies the petrosal and mastoid part of temporal bone, the internal auditory meatus, the jugular foramen and the sigmoid sinus.
- **Inferiorly** lies the occipital bone, foramen magnum and hypoglossal canal.

- The fossa is covered **superiorly** by the tentorium cerebelli.

CONTENTS

The *cerebellum* lies posterior to the brainstem and consists of two hemispheres united in the midline by cerebellar vermis (Fig. 3.2). Three peduncles connect each hemisphere to the three parts of the brainstem. The superior peduncle enters the midbrain, the middle peduncle consists of transverse fibres of the pons and the inferior peduncle arises from the medulla. Blood supply is from:

1. posterior inferior cerebellar artery
2. anterior inferior cerebellar artery
3. superior cerebellar artery.

The *pons* lies anterior to the cerebellum and is continuous with the midbrain superiorly and with the medulla oblongata inferiorly. Beneath the floor of the

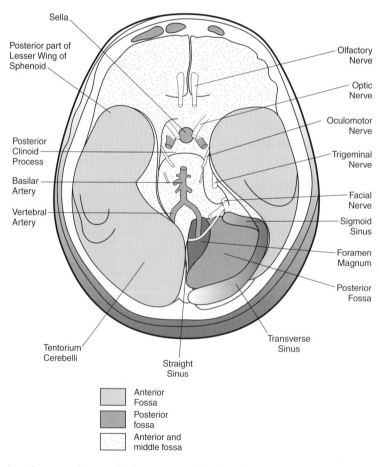

Figure 3.1   Relationship of posterior fossa with other intracranial landmarks

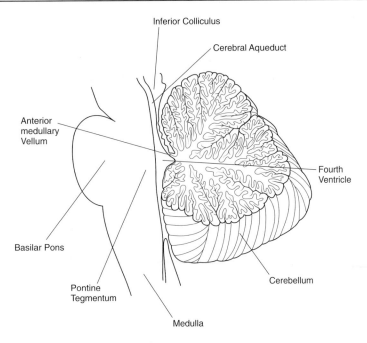

Figure 3.2   Saggital view of contents of the posterior fossa

fourth ventricle the pons contains the nuclei of CN V (sensory and motor), VI, VII and part of VIII. Blood supply is from the pontine branches of the basilar artery.

The *medulla oblongata* is piriform in shape and extends from the lower margin of the pons to a transverse plane passing above the first pair of cervical nerves. It contains the nuclei of CN IX, X, XI and XII. Blood supply anteriorly is via the vertebral and basilar arteries and laterally and posteriorly by posterior inferior cerebellar arteries.

The *fourth ventricle* – the substance of the midbrain surrounds the cerebral aqueduct and the substance of the lower medulla surrounds the central canal. Between the two, however, the substance of the pons and the upper medulla lies anteriorly and the central canal is expanded as the fourth ventricle. It is tent-shaped and situated anterior to the cerebellum. It has three apertures, one median (foramen of Magendie) and two lateral (foramina of Luschka) through which CSF escapes from the ventricular system into subarachnoid space for absorption by the arachnoid villi.

The arteries in the posterior cranial fossa comprise the two vertebral and the basilar arteries with their branches (Fig. 3.1).

The vertebral artery runs forward in front of the ligamentum denticulatum between the lower rootlets of the hypoglossal nerve and the upper rootlets of the first cervical nerve. It gives off the anterior spinal artery and the posterior inferior cerebellar artery and spirals up to meet its opposite fellow at the lower border of the pons to form the basilar artery.

The basilar artery runs up the front of the pons and ends at the upper border of the pons by branching on each side into superior cerebellar and posterior cerebral arteries.

The veins of the posterior fossa drain the cerebellum and brainstem. The major venous structures include:

1. the venous sinuses (straight, lateral, occipital, superior petrosal, left and right transverse)
2. great vein of Galen
3. petrosal vein.

The posterior fossa contains four foraminae:

1. The *foramen magnum* contains the medulla oblongata, which becomes the spinal cord
2. The *hypoglossal canal* which contains CN XII
3. The *jugular foramen* contains the sigmoid sinus, which becomes the internal jugular vein, CN IX, X, XI
4. The *internal auditory meatus* transmits CN VII, VIII and the nervus intermedius.

KEY POINTS

- The posterior fossa contains the cerebellum and brainstem
- The fourth ventricle lies between the cerebellum and brainstem
- Cranial nerves IV–XII are either transmitted or contained within the posterior fossa
- The veins in the posterior fossa may contribute to intraoperative complications such as haemorrhage, haematoma or venous air embolism
- Increased volume in the posterior fossa may lead to brainstem ischaemia.

FURTHER READING

Neurology. In: Gray's Anatomy, 35th edn. Warwick R, Williams P (eds). Longman, Edinburgh 1973, pp. 260–278

Last RJ. Anatomy: regional and applied. Churchill Livingstone, London 1972, pp. 760–763

4

NERVES: ANATOMY AND FUNCTION

S. Gupta

INTRODUCTION

Neurones are the basic building blocks of the nervous system and are involved in the integration and transmission of nerve impulses. A typical motor neurone and sensory neurone are shown in Figure 4.1 and 4.2 respectively. The axon acquires a sheath of myelin, a protein-lipid complex made up of many layers of the cell membranes of Schwann cells. In the CNS of mammals, more neurones are myelinated, but the cells that form the myelin are oligodendrocytes rather than Schwann cells.

From the *functional* point of view the neurones generally have four important zones (Fig. 4.1).

1. A receptor or dendritic zone where multiple local potential changes generated by the synaptic connections are integrated.
2. A site where propagated action potentials are generated (the initial segment in the spinal motor

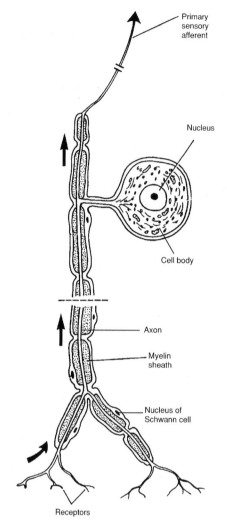

Figure 4.2   A sensory neurone with cell body, bifurcating axon and peripheral and central connections

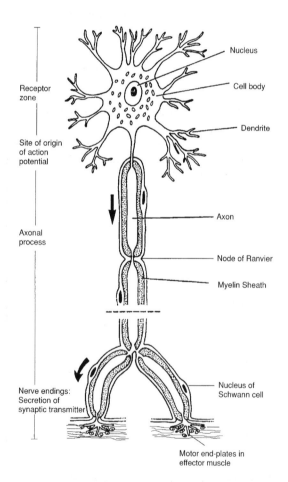

Figure 4.1   A motor neurone with myelinated axon. The four functional zones of the neurone are labelled to the left

neurone, the initial node of Ranvier in the cutaneous sensory neurone).
3. An axonal process that transmits propagated impulses to the nerve endings.
4. The nerve endings, where action potentials cause the release of synaptic transmitters. The cell body is often located in the dendritic zone end of the axon.

All necessary proteins are synthesised in the endoplasmic reticulum and Golgi apparatus of the cell body and then transported along the axon to the synaptic knobs by the process of axoplasmic flow. Thus, the cell body maintains the functional and anatomic integrity of the axon; if the axon is cut, the part distal to the cut degenerates (Wallerian degeneration). Most of the energy requirement of a neurone is supplied by the

Na$^+$/K$^+$ATPase and this maintains membrane polarisation. During maximal activity, the energy requirement rate is doubled.

Nerve cells are stimulated by electrical, chemical and mechanical stimuli. When an adequate stimulus is applied, the propagated nerve impulse is known as an action potential which is normally conducted along the axon to its termination. The action potential is an 'all or none' phenomena (Fig. 4.3). If the stimulus is subthreshold in intensity, no action potential is generated. With adequate stimulus, the action potential occurs with a constant amplitude and form regardless of the strength of the stimulus.

Saltatory conduction occurs in faster conducting myelinated nerves where depolarisation jumps from one node of Ranvier to the next. Nerve fibres are classified (see Table 4.1) depending on diameter and conduction velocity. The relative susceptibility of mammalian A, B and C nerve fibres to conduction block produced by various agents is shown in Table 4.1.

KEY POINTS

- Neurones are the building blocks of the nervous system. The motor and sensory neurones are different as shown in Figures 4.1 and 4.2.

- The cell body maintains the functional and anatomical integrity of the neurone.
- A neurone may be divided into four zones: receptor zone, zone where conducted impulses originate, axonal zone and the nerve endings where synaptic transmitters are released.

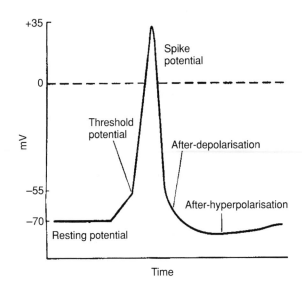

Figure 4.3   A typical action potential in a neurone

Fibre type	Function	Fibre diameter (mm)	Conduction velocity (m/s)	Hypoxia	Pressure	LA
Aα	Proprioception; Somatic motor	12–20	70–120	++	+++	+
Aβ	Touch, pressure	2–12	30–70			
Aγ	Motor to muscle spindle	3–6	15–30			
Aδ	Pain, cold, touch	2–5	12–30			
B	Preganglionic autonomic	< 3	3–15	+++	++	+
C Dorsal root	Pain, temperature, mechanoreception, reflex response	0.4–1.2	0.5–2	++	++	+++
C Sympathetic	Postganglionic sympathetics	0.3–1.3	0.7–2.3			

Table 4.1 Mammalian nerve fibre types and their susceptibility to conduction blockade by hypoxia, pressure and local anaesthetics

A and B fibres are myelinated; C fibres are unmyelinated; LA = local anaesthetic; + = least susceptible; ++ = intermediate susceptibility; +++ = most susceptible

- A minimum threshold stimulus is necessary to initiate a propagated action potential (Fig. 4.3) which is an 'all or none' phenomena.

FURTHER READING

Ganong WF. Review of medical physiology. Excitable tissue: nerve. Stamford, Connecticut: Appleton & Lange, 1997, pp. 47–59

Section 2

PHYSIOLOGY

5

CEREBRAL BLOOD FLOW

M. Prabhu, A.K. Gupta

INTRODUCTION

Although the adult brain constitutes only 2% of body mass, it accounts for 20% of basal oxygen consumption (50 ml/min). Mean resting cerebral blood flow (CBF) in adults is about 50 ml/100 g/min. The anatomy of the cerebral circulation is described in Chapter 2.

The whole brain oxygen consumption is approximately 3.5 ml of oxygen/100 g of brain tissue/min. The substantial demands for both oxygen and glucose are met by maintaining CBF. CBF is related to cerebral perfusion pressure (CPP) and cerebrovascular resistance (CVR) as follows:

CBF = CPP / CVR where

CPP = Mean arterial pressure (MAP) – Intracranial pressure (ICP) – venous pressure (VP).

REGULATION OF CBF

Factors affecting CBF are shown in Figure 5.1.

Myogenic Regulation (Autoregulation)

Autoregulation is defined as the maintenance of a constant level of CBF in the presence of alterations in the perfusion pressure. The normal physiological limits of autoregulation are approximately 50 mmHg and 150 mmHg (mean arterial pressure). These limits are in reality less distinct than shown in Figure 5.1. Autoregulation is brought about by changes in CVR caused by myogenic reflexes in the resistance vessels probably due to changes in transmural tension.

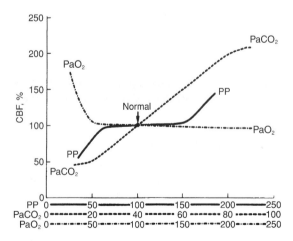

Figure 5.1   Factors affecting CBF: PP = perfusion pressure (mmHg), $PaCO_2$ = arterial carbon dioxide tension (mmHg), PaO_2 = arterial oxygen tension (mmHg)

Autoregulation changes in the presence of intracranial pathology and volatile anaesthetic agents (see Chapter 9). Chronic hypertension or sympathetic activation shifts the autoregulatory curve to the right.

Flow-Metabolism Coupling

Increased neuronal activity causes an increase in cerebral metabolic rate (CMR), resulting in a well matched increase in CBF. The parallel change in CBF with CMR is known as 'flow-metabolism coupling'. Acetylcholine, nitric oxide, serotonin and substance P have been described as mediators but the precise mechanism of this coupling is still unknown. There is evidence to suggest that CBF may be modulated by changes in glucose consumption rather than O_2 consumption.

Chemical Regulation

Arterial carbon dioxide tension (PaCO2)

CO_2 is a potent vasodilator. CBF changes by 1–2 ml/100 g/min for each 1 mmHg change in $PaCO_2$ within physiological limits. These changes are believed to be driven by changes in extracellular or interstitial H^+ concentration. However, after 6–8 hours, the CBF returns to baseline values because CSF pH gradually normalises as a result of the extrusion of bicarbonate.

Arterial oxygen tension

Although arterial oxygen was previously not thought to effect CBF unless PaO_2 fell below 50 mmHg recent evidence from studies in human volunteers have demonstrated the threshold for hypoxic vasodilatation exists at arterial saturations of 90–92%. Localised hypoxia may cause vasodilatation and an increase in CBF.

Potassium and adenosine

Both potassium and adenosine are potent vasodilators. Increased concentrations are detected during seizures, direct cortical stimulation and hypoxia which causes an increase in CBF.

Calcium is a potent vasoconstrictor in high concentrations. Some calcium antagonists blunt hypoxic vasodilatation and prevent adenosine release.

Recent evidence suggests that nitric oxide (NO) plays an important role in cerebral vasodilatation caused by hypercapnia, ischaemia, increased cerebral metabolic rate, excitatory amino acids and volatile anaesthetic agents.

Neurogenic regulation

The autonomic nervous system mainly affects the larger cerebral vessels. β-1 adrenergic stimulation results in vasodilatation, whereas α-2 adrenergic stimulation causes vasoconstriction. Significant vaso-constriction can be produced by extremely high concentration of catecholamines as in haemorrhagic shock.

Blood viscosity

CBF can be influenced by blood viscosity, of which haematocrit is the single most important determinant. Studies suggest that a haematocrit of 30–34% may result in optimal oxygen delivery. However, if maximum vasodilatation already exists, O_2 delivery may decrease with haemodilution.

EFFECT OF ANAESTHETIC AGENTS ON CBF (see also Chapters 8–10)

Inhalational Agents

All volatile anaesthetic agents produce a dose-related decrease in CMR while causing an increase in CBF. Flow and metabolism is not actually uncoupled, but the gradient of the slope is increased with higher doses of agent. Nitrous oxide (N_2O) may cause an increase in CBF without a decrease in CMR. This increase is unaffected by hypocapnia.

Intravenous Agents

Thiopentone, etomidate and propofol all cause a reduction in global CMR and CBF. Even high doses of thiopentone or propofol do not affect autoregulation, flow-metabolism coupling or CO_2 responsiveness.

Opiates

The general pattern is one of modest reduction in both CMR and CBF. High doses of morphine (3 mg/kg) and moderate doses of fentanyl (15 μg/kg) have little effect on CBF and CMR. High doses of fentanyl (50–100 μg/kg) and sufentanyl (10 μg/kg) depress CMR and CBF. Alfentanil (0.3 μg/kg) shows no reduction in CBF.

OTHER DRUGS

Benzodiazepines cause reduction in CMR and CBF by about 20–25%. Ketamine increases in CMR, CBF and ICP. These changes can be partially attenuated by hypocapnia. Lidocaine produces a dose-related reduction in $CMRO_2$. Non-depolarising neuromuscular blockers have little effect on CBF and CMR. Succinylcholine can produce ICP increases, probably secondary to rise in CBF. However, these changes are transient and mild.

MEASUREMENT OF CBF

Methods of measuring CBF can be *regional* or *global*. All methods that provide an absolute estimate of CBF use one of two principles. They either measure the distribution of a tracer or estimate regional CBF (rCBF) from a washin or washout curve of an indicator. Other techniques measure a related flow variable (arterial flow velocity) or infer changes in flow from changes in metabolic parameters.

Kety Schmidt Technique

Nitrous oxide (10–15%) is inhaled and arterial and jugular venous samples are obtained at rapid intervals for measurement of N_2O levels. Plotting concentration against time produces a rapid rise in *arterial* N_2O concentration and a slower *venous* rise. The rate of equilibration of the two curves measured reflects the rate at which N_2O is being delivered thereby giving an estimate of global CBF. Actual CBF is proportional to the area between the arterial and venous curves.

Xenon-133 Washout Technique

This technique measures regional CBF. Radioactive Xenon is inhaled or injected into the carotid artery or the aorta and a washout curve is obtained. Individual washout curves can be separated into high and slow washout components which may represent flow in grey and white matter. This method primarily estimates cortical blood flow.

Tomographic rCBF Measurement

Dynamic CT

Rapid sequential computed tomography (CT) may be used to quantify the washout of a radioactive contrast agent.

Single photon emission computed tomography (SPECT)

This technique uses gamma emitting and positron emitting isotopes respectively, to produce tomographic images of regional CBF.

Functional magnetic resonance imaging (f MRI)

An intravenous MR contrast agent can give a reflection of CBF. Changes in MR signal intensity produced by decreases in regional deoxyhaemoglobin levels can give tomographic images of changes in regional CBF.

Indirect or Non-quantitative Measures

1. Doppler ultrasonography: Provides an indirect measure of arterial flow velocity.
2. Magnetic resonance spectroscopy (MRS): Provides information regarding intracellular pH and tissue levels of adenosine triphosphate and lactate.
3. Near infrared spectroscopy (NIRS): measures regional haemoglobin oxygenation and cytochrome redox state (see Chapter 54).
4. Laser Doppler flowmetry (LDF): An investigational technique measuring the Doppler shift of reflected laser light induced by movement of red blood cells within the microcirculation. Provides a non-quantitative measurement of microvascular blood flow in a small area of tissue.
5. Thermal dilution flow probes: These are also investigational and consist of a flexible cortical strip electrode for placement on the brain at craniotomy which provides information on relative, not absolute, changes in CBF in a relatively small (20–30 mm^3) volume of brain.

KEY POINTS

- The brain is highly metabolic and has a high blood flow.
- Five major factors control CBF: $PaCO_2$, autoregulation, PaO_2 flow-metabolism coupling and the autonomic nervous system.
- Similar factors control CBF and CBV.
- Inhalational agents are potent vasodilators.
- By decreasing CMR, intravenous anaesthetic agents reduce CBF and CBV.

FURTHER READING

Menon DK. Cerebral circulation. In: Cardiovascular physiology. London: BMJ Publishing Group, 1995

Strong A, Pollay M. Cerebral blood flow. In: The practice of neurosurgery, Vol 1. Baltimore: Williams & Wilkins, 1996

Todd MM, Warner DS. Neuroanesthesia: a critical review. In: Rogers MC, Tinker JH, Covino BG, Longnecker DE (eds) Principles and practice of anesthesiology. Chicago: Mosby-Year Book, 1993, pp. 1599–1648

6

INTRACRANIAL PRESSURE

M. Prabhu, A.K. Gupta

Intracranial pressure is the pressure inside the cranial vault relative to atmospheric pressure.

PATHOPHYSIOLOGY

The rigid cranium surrounding the brain creates a unique protective space. As brain tissue is nearly incompressible, any rise in pressure will cause CSF and blood to be expressed out of the cranium. Thus change in volume of one compartment is accompanied by a reciprocal change in another compartment.

The intracranial contents can be divided into four compartments:

- Solid material ≈ 10%;
- Tissue water ≈ 75%;
- CSF (150 ml) ≈ 10%;
- Blood (50–75 ml) ≈ 5%.

MONRO KELLY DOCTRINE

Raised ICP causes brain damage by reducing CPP or by focal compression of brain tissue due to distortion and herniation of intracranial contents.

CONTROL OF ICP

VOLUME BUFFERING (PRESSURE–VOLUME RELATIONSHIP)

The pressure–volume relationship is given in Figure 6.1. During initial compensation, between points 1 and 2, there is hardly any rise in ICP with changes in intracranial volume. At point 2, further increases

in volume cause a slight rise in ICP. As volume increases, there is a steady decline in compliance which increases the ICP even more (point 3) until a small rise in volume is associated with a marked rise in ICP causing a fall in the perfusion pressure and ultimately cerebral ischaemia (between points 3 and 4).

CSF

The reduction of the volume from one compartment as a result of an increase in another compartment is known as 'spatial compensation'. CSF plays the biggest role in spatial compensation. As a space-occupying lesion expands, it will cause progressive reduction of the CSF space (reduced size of the ventricles/ basal cisterns). Rapidly growing masses (e.g. haematoma) exhaust spatial compensation quickly resulting in a rapid rise of ICP.

Cerebral blood volume (CBV)

Most of the intracranial blood volume is contained in the venous sinuses and pial veins. This acts as a buffer in the event of raised ICP. Factors affecting CBV include:

- *Venous distension* – from jugular venous obstruction, increased intrathoracic pressure, raised central venous pressure, head down tilt, vasodilators.
- *$PaCO_2$* – Both CBF and CBV increase with raised $PaCO_2$, but the CBV response curve is flatter than the CBF curve (Fig. 6.2). A reduction in $PaCO_2$ from 40–20 mmHg (5.3–2.7 kPa) results in a 65% reduction in CBF but only a 28% reduction in CBV (2.8 ml/100 g). This small change in

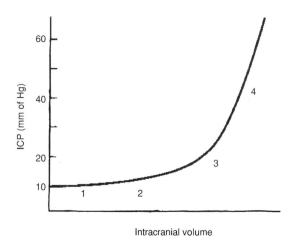

Figure 6.1   Intracranial pressure volume curve

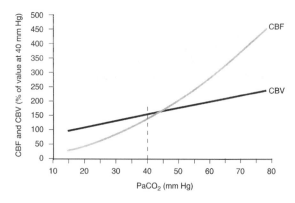

Figure 6.2   Relationship of cerebral blood flow and blood volume with changes in arterial carbon dioxide. (Adapted with permission from Todd MM, Warner DS. Neuro-anesthesia: a critical review.)

intracranial volume will have a significant reduction in ICP in the presence of intracranial hypertension because the system operates on the steep part of the pressure volume curve (see Fig. 6.1).

- *PaO₂* – Cerebral vasodilatation occurs with hypoxia resulting in a rise in CBV. There is evidence that hyperoxia causes vasoconstriction although there is no human evidence to suggest this is clinically significant.
- *Flow-metabolism coupling* (see Chapter 5) – Increased metabolic demand increases CBF, CBV and ICP.
- *Autoregulation* (see Chapter 5) – A fall in MAP can lead to a decrease in cerebrovascular tone causing cerebral vasodilatation and increase in CBV within limits.

CLINICAL FEATURES OF RAISED ICP

There are no pathognomonic signs or symptoms of raised ICP. Most of them are related to traction and distortion of pain-sensitive cerebral blood vessels and dura mater. Pressure headaches seen on waking up and relieved by vomiting, papilloedema, amaurosis fugax (intermittent loss of vision), unilateral pupillary dilation, oculomotor or abducent nerve palsy and finally loss of consciousness and respiratory depression all feature with increasing pressure.

The oval pupil is an important sign and represents a transitional stage between the normal and fixed, unreactive pupil.

RADIOLOGICAL SIGNS (see Chapter 65)

1. Skull X-rays
   - In children up to the age of 8–9 years, diastasis of sutures, erosion of the dorsum sellae and thinning of the vault may be present.
   - In adults, erosion of the dorsum sellae, displaced

pineal gland, bony erosion and abnormal calcification may indicate chronic intracranial hypertension.

2. CT
   - A CT scan may show a mass (e.g. haematoma or tumour), hydrocephalus or brain swelling. The signs of raised ICP include midline shift, obliteration of the CSF cisterns around the brainstem, effacement of the ventricles and cortical sulci.
3. MRI
   - MRI is useful in demonstrating midline and posterior fossa structures. MRI is more expensive, slower and requires more patient cooperation.

MONITORING ICP (see Chapter 52)

KEY POINTS

- The intracranial contents are enclosed in a rigid cranial vault.
- Raised ICP causes secondary brain injury.
- Changes to the CSF space is a major compensatory factor with raised ICP.
- Manipulation of CBV can rapidly reduce ICP if intracranial hypertension exists.
- CBV does not change in parallel with CBF.

FURTHER READING

Lee KR, Hoff JT. Intracranial pressure. In: Youmans neurological surgery. London: WB Saunders, 1996, pp. 491–519

Shalmon E, Caron M, Becker D. Intracranial pathology and pathophysiology. In: Tindall GT, Cooper PR, Barrow DL (eds) The practice of neurosurgery. Baltimore: Williams & Wilkins, 1996, pp. 45–70

Todd MM, Warner DS. Neuroanesthesia: a critical review. In: Rogers MC, Tinker JH, Covino BG, Longnecker DE (eds) Principles and practice of anesthesiology. St Louis: Mosby-Year Book, 1993, pp. 1599–1648

7

CEREBROSPINAL FLUID

J. Coles

INTRODUCTION

Cerebrospinal fluid is contained within the sub-arachnoid space, surrounding the brain and spinal cord, lying between the pia mater (which is closely adherent to the underlying neural tissue) and the arachnoid mater.

STRUCTURE AND FUNCTION

The majority of the 450–500 ml of CSF produced daily is formed in the choroid plexus of the ventricles. The CSF circulates around the brain and spinal cord through the ventricular system and subarachnoid space (Fig. 7.1). The two lateral ventricles communicate with the third ventricle through the foramen of Munro, which communicates with the fourth ventricle via the aqueduct of Sylvius. From here fluid is free to circulate around the brainstem and spinal cord, cerebellum and cerebral hemispheres. There is about 150 ml of fluid circulating around the adult central nervous system, which is constantly produced by the choroid plexus and absorbed through the arachnoid villi into the dural venous sinus network. CSF acts both as a supporting fluid cushion for the intracranial contents and as an important pathway for nutrients and chemical mediators.

SECRETION AND COMPOSITION

CSF is a clear colourless fluid formed as an ultrafiltrate of plasma and is composed of 99% water with a specific gravity of 1.004–1.007. The normal pressure which may be expressed using Davson's equation: *(resistance to csf outflow)* $^\times$ *(CSF formation rate)* + *(pressure in sagittal sinus)* ranges from 80 to 180 mm of CSF (< 10 mmHg). It has a composition similar to plasma (Table 7.1).

Hypocapnia, hypothermia, high serum osmolality and alkalosis (metabolic or respiratory) can all reduce CSF production. Many agents acting as inhibitors of ion transport, including acetazolamide, digoxin, amiloride, furosemide, bumetanide, omeprazole, cholera toxin, norepinephrine, angiotensin II, 5-hydroxytryptamine and some vasoactive peptides have also been shown to inhibit CSF formation.

Anaesthetic agents have varying effects on CSF production and reabsorption. The intravenous anaesthetic agents propofol, thiopentone and etomidate and fentanyl have no significant effect on the rate of CSF formation or absorption. The volatile agents, in contrast, have varied but more significant effects. Isoflurane is the only agent which reduces CSF production and facilitates reabsorption. Desflurane induces an increase in CSF production, whilst enflurane combines the deleterious effects of increasing production and reducing absorption. The other inhalational agents, halothane and sevoflurane, decrease CSF production but may also decrease its absorption.

The total white blood cell (WBC) count in normal adult CSF is 0–5 per mm^3 (lymphocytes and mono-

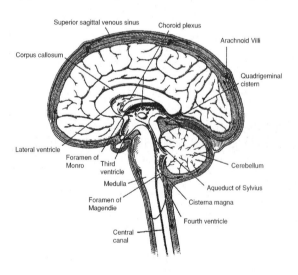

Figure 7.1   Circulation of cerebral spinal fluid. (Modified and reproduced, with permission, from Meyer FB. Cerebrospinal fluid physiology and the management of increased intracranial pressure. Mayo Clin Pro 1990; 65: 687.)

Table 7.1 Comparison of CSF and Plasma (Modified and reproduced, with permission, from Ganong WF.		
Substance	CSF	Plasma
Na$^+$ (meq/Kg H$_2$O)	147	150
K$^+$ (meq/Kg H$_2$O)	2.9	4.6
Mg^{2+} (meq/Kg H$_2$O)	2.2	1.6
Ca^{2+} (meq/Kg H$_2$O)	2.3	4.7
Cl$^-$ (meq/Kg H$_2$O)	113	99
HCO$_3^-$ (meq/Kg H$_2$O)	25.1	24.8
pCO$_2$ (kPa)	6.6	5.3
pH	7.33	7.4
Osmolality (mosm/Kg H$_2$O)	289	289
Protein (g/l)	0.2	60
Glucose (mmol/l)	3.6	5.6

cytes), and even one granulocyte is considered abnormal. To the naked eye the normally clear CSF will appear cloudy when there are greater than 200 white blood cells per mm^3 or 400 red blood cells per mm^3. The typical changes in CSF microscopy in meningitis and neuromuscular conditions such as multiple sclerosis are displayed in Table 7.2.

In subarachnoid haemorrhage a yellow discolouration of CSF following centrifugation is a diagnostic sign. This xanthochromia, appears several hours following an acute bleed and is due to haemolysis of red blood cells. It is maximal at 1 week and usually disappears after 3 weeks. It can be distinguished from a 'bloody tap', which does not clear as the CSF drains from the puncture needle. A CT scan is the diagnostic tool of choice for identifying subarachnoid haemorrhage.

KEY POINTS

- CSF is an ultrafiltrate of plasma.
- Approx 150 ml circulates around the CNS in adults.
- Normal pressure < 10 mmHg.

- Production and absorption can be affected by many factors.
- Examination of CSF can aid in diagnosis of certain conditions.

FURTHER READING

Artu AA. Isoflurane does not increase the rate of CSF production in the dog. Anesthesiology 1984; 60: 193–197

Artu AA. Effects of enflurane and isoflurane on resistance to reabsorption of cerebrospinal fluid in dogs. Anesthesiology 1984; 61: 529–533

Artu AA. Propofol combined with halothane or with fentanyl/halothane does not alter the rate of CSF formation or resistance to reabsorption of CSF in rabbits. Journal of Neurosurgical Anesthesiology 1993; 5(4): 250–257

Dougherty JM, Roth RM. Cerebral spinal fluid. Emergency medicine clinics of North America 1986; 4(2): 281–297

Kazemi H, Johnson DC. Regulation of cerebrospinal fluid acid-base balance. Physiological Reviews 1986; 66(4): 953–1037

Segal MB. Extracellular and cerebrospinal fluids. Journal of Inherited Metabolic Disease 1993; 16: 617–638

Table 7.2 Cerebrospinal fluid findings in some common disorders.
Traumatic tap correction: For every 1000 red cells/mm^3 subtract one white cell/mm^3.

CSF	Normal	Meningitis Bacterial	Viral	Tuberculous	Multiple sclerosis
Appearance	Clear and colourless	Turbid	Clear to turbid	Turbid	Clear
Cell count/mm^3	0–5	> 1000	< 500	< 500	5–60
Cell type	Lymphocytes	Polymorphs	Lymphocytes	Lymphocytes	Monocytes
Protein concentration (g/L)	0.15–0.45	> 1.5	0.5–1.0	1–5	0.4–1.0
CSF glucose	At least 50% of blood level	Less than 50% of blood level	At least 50% of blood level	Less than 50% of blood level	At least 50% of blood level
Ig	< 15% of protein				> 15% of protein
Oligoclonal IgG	None				Bands present in 80%

Section 3
PHARMACOLOGY

8

INTRAVENOUS ANAESTHETIC AGENTS

J. Coles, A.K. Gupta

INTRODUCTION

There are certain properties that the 'ideal' intravenous agent for use during neuroanaesthesia and neurocritical care should possess:

- Rapid recovery of consciousness to enable early neurological assessment.
- Easily and rapidly titratable.
- Minimal effects on other systems, e.g. cardiovascular, respiratory, renal, hepatic.
- Analgesia.
- Favourable effect on cerebral haemodynamics:
  - A reduction in CMR coupled with CBF.
  - No increase in CBV.
  - Vasoreactivity to CO_2 maintained.
  - Cerebrovascular autoregulation maintained.
- Does not predispose to seizures.

Propofol, thiopentone, and etomidate are the agents most commonly used for intravenous induction of anaesthesia for neurosurgery.

PROPOFOL

Propofol provides smooth induction of anaesthesia with few excitatory side-effects. It produces a progressive reduction in CBF coupled with global metabolic suppression with up to 60% reduction in $CMRO_2$. Intracranial pressure may be reduced, particularly in patients with an elevated baseline ICP. However, it can cause a dose-dependent reduction in arterial pressure and compromise CPP. The responsiveness of the cerebral circulation to CO_2 and autoregulation is maintained with propofol. As well as these beneficial effects on cerebral haemodynamics propofol has free radical scavanging properties which are greater than thiopentone, and *in vitro* has calcium channel blocking and glutamate antagonist properties.

The effects on the electroencephalogram (EEG) include a dose-related suppression of activity in the β-frequency range and increases in the δ range, followed by an isoelectric EEG. It is an anticonvulsant, however seizure activity has been anecdotally reported. The effect on electrically stimulated motor evoked potentials and somatosensory evoked potentials is dose-dependent and low dose infusions are useful during procedures requiring intraoperative neurophysiological monitoring. Propofol has been used successfully for conscious sedation during awake craniotomy.

BARBITURATES

Thiopentone is the only drug with evidence of protection in focal ischaemia, and is also of proven cerebral protection during cardiac surgery. It may be useful during periods of temporary intraoperative ischaemia (dose ≥ 5 mg/kg) if hypotension can be avoided. It is less protective in global compared to focal ischaemia. It also has significant free radical scavenging properties, reduces calcium influx, and may block sodium channels. A coupled decrease in CBF occurs with $CMRO_2$. If coupling is disrupted, CBF may increase.

EEG effects include initial fast activity anteriorly followed by slowing leading to burst suppression with infusions doses up to 15 mg/kg/h after an initial loading dose. When $CMRO_2$ is reduced by 50%, the EEG becomes isoelectric and increasing the dose has no further effect on $CMRO_2$ or CBF. The effect on evoked potentials is also dose-dependent ($\uparrow$ latency, $\downarrow$ amplitude).

Prolonged infusion is useful in status epilepticus and refractory intracranial hypertension, and can be titrated to burst suppression. After prolonged infusion, thiopentone is associated with dilated pupils, a protracted recovery period and depression of consciousness.

Methohexitone has epileptogenic properties and may be useful for augmenting abnormal EEG activity during surgical treatment of focal epilepsy.

ETOMIDATE

Etomidate depresses the cardiovascular system minimally and is the agent of choice when preservation of CPP is crucial. The effect on $CMRO_2$ and CBF is similar to the barbiturates. It is a potent suppressant of corticosteroid synthesis which is evident after one induction dose. The clinical relevance of this is uncertain. Seizures can be elicited in susceptible patients with low-dose etomidate and it has been used to unmask seizure foci during operative EEG mapping for epilepsy surgery.

The effects on the EEG are similar to those of the barbiturates although an isoelectric EEG may be preceded by intermittent spike activity which may be associated with myoclonus. Etomidate has minimal effects on evoked potentials and may increase somatosensory evoked potentials.

KETAMINE

Ketamine increases global MAP, CBF and ICP with specific increases in regional CBF and $CMRO_2$ in limbic structures. These effects are partially reversible using induced hypocapnia and/or the administration of thiopentone or benzodiazepines.

Ketamine produces hypersynchronous δ waves in the EEG, but has little effect on somatosensory or motor evoked potentials.

Although ketamine may offer theoretical cerebral protection via NMDA antagonism, its use in neuroanaesthesia is limited by its ability to increase ICP.

BENZODIAZEPINES

All produce a small reduction in CBF, $CMRO_2$ and ICP whilst preserving cerebral autoregulation and vasoreactivity to CO_2. This effect is inconsistent and much less marked than the intravenous induction agents. A ceiling effect occurs whereby increasing doses do not produce greater reductions in these variables.

All are anticonvulsant and increase seizure threshold. All effects, including any reduction in ICP, are reversible using the competitive antagonist flumazenil, the use of which may precipitate seizures.

Midazolam produces a dose-related increase in high amplitude EEG activity below 8 Hz. Burst suppression does not occur, and the EEG does not appear to become isoelectric.

Prolonged sedation precludes these drugs as induction agents for neuroanaesthesia, although the short acting drugs are appropriate as premedicant agents.

KEY POINTS

- Propofol, thiopentone and etomidate have similar effects on cerebral haemodynamics and metabolism.
- All three agents reduce $CMRO_2$ and CBF and maintain responsiveness to CO_2 and autoregulation.
- These agents cause dose-dependent suppression of EEG. Burst suppression and isoelectric EEG can be achieved.
- Ketamine causes increased CBF and ICP, although it is an NMDA antagonist.
- Benzodiazepines have a small effect on blood flow and metabolism. They are anticonvulsant drugs but EEG burst suppression cannot be achieved.

FURTHER READING

Michenfelder JD. The interdependency of cerebral function and metabolic effects following maximum doses of thiopental in the dog. Anesthesiology 1974; 41: 231

Ravussin P, Guinard JP, Ralley F, Thorin D. Effect of propofol on cerebrospinal fluid pressure and cerebral perfusion pressure in patients undergoing craniotomy. Anaesthesia 1988; 43(suppl): 37–41

Ravussin P, Tempelhoff R, Modica P, Bayer-Merger MM. Propofol vs thiopental – isoflurane for neurosurgical anesthesia: comparison of hemodynamics, CSF pressure and recovery. J Neurosurg Anesthesiol 1991; 3: 85

Todd MM, Warner DS, Sokoll MD, et al. A prospective comparative trial of three anesthetics for elective supratentorial craniotomy. Propofol/fentanyl, isoflurane/nitrous oxide and fentanyl/nitrous oxide. Anesthesiology 1993; 78: 1005–1020

9

INHALATIONAL ANAESTHETIC AGENTS

J. Coles, A. Summors

GENERAL PRINCIPLES

All the fluorinated agents have effects on CBF, CBV and $CMRO_2$.

- CBF increases with all agents by a direct *intrinsic* effect which reduces arterial wall tension and results in cerebral vasodilatation. The magnitude of the increase in CBF depends on the balance between this *intrinsic* vasodilatory action and the reduction in blood flow secondary to a dose-related decrease in $CMRO_2$.
- The order of rise in CBF is approximately halothane > enflurane > isoflurane ≥ sevoflurane. Desflurane has similar effects to isoflurane.
- CBV increases as a consequence of vasodilatation, which in turn increases brain volume and possibly ICP.
- The gradient of the flow-metabolism coupling relationship increases in clinically used doses (see Fig. 9.1). These changes are attenuated by hypocapnia.
- CO_2 reduction attenuates the increase in CBF. The normal CO_2 *vs* CBF curve is shifted to the left. Hypercapnia causes a more rapid increase in CBF with these agents.
- Autoregulation of CBF is impaired in a dose-dependent manner until CBF becomes dependent on mean arterial pressure.
- Progressive slowing of the EEG at concentrations > 1 MAC.

ISOFLURANE

Isoflurane produces less cerebral vasodilatation than the other agents except possibly sevoflurane. Global

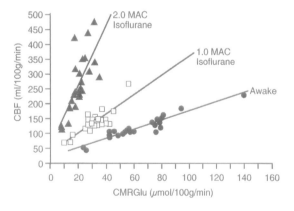

Figure 9.1 Changes in gradient of flow-metabolism coupling in an animal model exposed to 1 and 2 MAC isoflurane. CMRGlu = cerebral metabolic rate of glucose reflecting metabolic rate, CBF = cerebral blood flow. (Adapted from Todd MM, Warner DS. Neuroanesthesia. In: Principles and practice of anesthesia, 1993.)

$CMRO_2$ and CBF decreases in low doses and there is greater cortical metabolic suppression than halothane. At higher concentrations (≥ 2 MAC), an isoelectric EEG is achieved with a 50% decrease in $CMRO_2$. Autoregulation is disrupted ≥ 1.5 MAC and a dose-dependent rise in CBF and ICP occurs. These effects can be attenuated by hypocapnia commenced when isoflurane is introduced or modified by baseline physiology and other pharmacological agents. Isoflurane may decrease CSF production and decreases its resistance to absorption.

SEVOFLURANE

Although similar to isoflurane in its cerebral vascular effects in animals, there is some evidence to suggest that it produces less intrinsic vasodilation of cerebral vessels and allows cerebral autoregulation to occur at higher anaesthetic concentrations compared with other agents. Up to 1.5 MAC sevoflurane anaesthesia causes little increase in ICP. The responsiveness of CBF to changes in $PaCO_2$ is also maintained. The lower blood:gas solubility coefficient (0.6) allows a rapid induction and recovery from anaesthesia and this combined with lower airway irritability has favoured its use for inhalation induction especially in children. The EEG is activated in some animal models and decreased in others.

HALOTHANE

Halothane has a potent vasodilatory action and produces a dose-related decrease in $CMRO_2$. However, the effect on $CMRO_2$ is less than with other agents and global CBF increases more than with equipotent concentrations of other inhalational agents. Unlike isoflurane, this rise in CBF can only be attenuated by hypocapnia if induced before addition of halothane. In concentrations above 2.5% there is evidence that it may be directly toxic on oxidative phosphorylation.

DESFLURANE

Cerebral effects are similar to isoflurane with a dose-dependent decrease in $CMRO_2$, CBF and loss of cerebral autoregulation. Under conditions of maximal metabolic suppression (high dose), intrinsic vasodilatation is also similar to isoflurane. Again these changes can be attenuated by hypocapnia induced at the time desflurane is commenced. During prolonged desflurane administration a slow increase in ICP is observed, possibly due to an increase in CSF production. EEG burst suppression is attenuated over time in some animal models.

ENFLURANE

Low concentrations decrease $CMRO_2$, CBF and cerebral autoregulation. Concentrations >1.5 MAC produce spike and wave EEG appearances especially with concomitant hypocapnia (< 4.0 kPa). The rate of production and resistance to reabsorption of CSF are also increased by enflurane, thereby exacerbating any increase in ICP.

NITROUS OXIDE

N_2O alone causes an increase in CBF without a decrease in $CMRO_2$. This increase is unaffected by hypocapnia alone but is modified when hypocapnia is combined with other inhalational agents or barbiturates. This may be of concern in cerebral ischaemia and should be used with care if ICP is raised.

Work in humans has shown N_2O to cause a significant increase in cerebral blood flow acting synergistically with inhalational agents. More importantly, the increase in CBF due to a combination of isoflurane and N_2O is greater than equipotent concentrations of the inhalational agent alone. Increases in ICP have been demonstrated when N_2O is used for patients with intracranial tumours. However one study addressing short-term outcome found no difference when N_2O was used.

KEY POINTS

- All inhalational anaesthetic agents cause cerebral vasodilatation.
- All agents effect cerebral autoregulation.
- All agents decrease $CMRO_2$.
- These effects are dose-dependent and modified by hypocapnia.
- Flow metabolism coupling is maintained in low doses.

FURTHER READING

Amorim P. Nitrous oxide in neuroanaesthesia: an appraisal. Curr Opin Anaesthiol 1999; 12: 511–515

Artru AA, Lam AM, Johnson JO, Sperry RJ. Intracranial pressure, middle cerebral artery flow velocity, and plasma inorganic fluoride concentrations in neurosurgical patients receiving sevoflurane or isoflurane. Anesth Analg 1997; 85: 587–592

Gosslight K, Foster R, Colohan AR, Bedford RF. Isoflurane for neuroanesthesia: risk factors for increase in intracranial pressure. Anesthesiology 1985; 63: 533

Matta BF, Heath KJ, Tipping K, Summors AC. Direct cerebral vasodilatory effects of sevoflurane and isoflurane. Anesthesiology 1999; 91: 677–680

Ostapkovich ND, Baker K, Fogarty-Mack P, Sisti M, Young ML. Cerebral blood flow and CO_2 reactivity is similar during remifentanyl/N_2O and fentanyl/N_2O anesthesia. Anesthesiology 1998; 89: 358–363

10

OPIOIDS AND ADJUVANT DRUGS

K. Grixti, A.K. Gupta

OPIOIDS

The opioid analgesics most frequently used in neuro-anaesthesia in the UK are morphine, fentanyl and alfentanil. Outside the UK, sufentanil has been used successfully for elective intracranial procedures. More recently, remifentanil is being used as a substitute to these agents. The effects of these agents on cerebral physiology are similar.

CEREBRAL HAEMODYNAMICS

Although opioids have little effect in low doses, in high doses reduction in CMR and CBF have been reported. Remifentanil decreases cerebral blood flow in a regionally selective fashion. A rise in ICP has been reported with some agents (alfentanil in patients with tumours, morphine due to histamine release, sufentanil in head-injured patients). However, none of these reports demonstrated any clinical significance or effect on outcome. All opioids maintain autoregulation and CO_2 reactivity of the cerebral circulation.

EEG ACTIVITY

Opioid drugs generally slow down the EEG into the theta and delta wave activity though isoelectricity and burst suppression is not seen. However, high-dose opiates such as fentanyl at 200 µg/kg are known to cause convulsions in animals. It is also reported that opioids may trigger limbic system epileptiform activity in known epileptics. This does not preclude using opioids for epilepsy surgery. These drugs have no significant effect on somatosensory, motor and auditory evoked potentials.

SEDATION AND EMERGENCE POSTOPERATIVELY

When combined with N_2O or propofol, opioids allow for more rapid emergence from anaesthesia than inhalational anaesthetics as sole agents. Remifentanil in turn allows an even more rapid emergence when compared with fentanyl and alfentanil due to a short half-life with plasma cholinesterase metabolism.

Hypocapnia-induced cerebral vasoconstriction may cause prolonged emergence due to an increased volume of distribution and a longer elimination. This is secondary to decreased cerebral blood flow causing a decrease in washout of the drug. A change in the drug lipid/plasma distribution coefficient due to a higher pH may also contribute.

CSF CIRCULATION

At low doses, fentanyl, sufentanil and alfentanil increase CSF absorption at the arachnoid villi. Fentanyl at high doses decreases the rate of CSF secretion and, along with sufentanil, may increase resistance to absorption.

OTHER EFFECTS

The responsiveness to carbon dioxide is decreased although hypoxic stimulation is preserved. The hypercapnic vasodilatation that can occur from opioid-induced respiratory depression may increase ICP if ventilation is not supported. This, together with hypoxia, can cause problems post-craniotomy especially in the elderly, diabetics and the obese.

Stimulation of the 5HT3 and dopamine receptors in the chemoreceptor trigger zone causes nausea and vomiting. Depression of the cough reflex caused may be detrimental postoperatively if brainstem reflexes are already impaired.

NALOXONE

It has been shown that naloxone alone probably has no important effect on CBF/CMR, and in narcotised patients these parameters are normalised with careful titration. However, abrupt naloxone reversal has resulted in hypertension, arrhythmias, myocardial ischaemia and intracranial haemorrhage.

NEUROMUSCULAR BLOCKING AGENTS

Coughing, straining and intolerance of the endotracheal tube can cause substantial increases in ICP, which can be avoided by the administration of neuromuscular blocking agents.

Suxamethonium can increase ICP and CBF due to muscle spindle activation. These increases are transient, clinically insignificant and can be avoided by 'precurarisation' if deemed necessary. Suxamethonium is not contraindicated in neurosurgical patients, particularly when the airway needs to be secured rapidly.

All *non-depolarising agents* have little effect on CBF or CMR. Only d-tubocurarine through the release of histamine can increase CBV and ICP. Atracurium has no significant effect and its level of histamine release is significantly less than d-tubocurarine. Atracurium does not accumulate and is suitable for use as a prolonged infusion. Laudanosine, a metabolite of atracurium, can cross the blood–brain barrier and predispose to seizures. However, even after prolonged infusion the serum levels of laudanosine are not clinically relevant.

Interactions with anticonvulsants, particularly phenytoin, shifts the dose–response curve for most relaxants to the right, thereby increasing dose requirements. The exception to this is atracurium which is independent of liver metabolism.

ANTIHYPERTENSIVES

SNP, GTN, hydralazine – Direct smooth muscle relaxation of the cerebral vasculature causes an increase in CBV and consequent rise in ICP. This change is independent of CBF which appears not to rise. The rise in CBV and ICP may be related to speed of infusion and the ability of compensatory mechanisms to take effect. This is demonstrated by the observation that hydralazine, which has a gradual onset of activity thus allowing spatial compensation, has least effect on ICP.

α and β blockers appear to have little or no effect on ICP/CBF. Labetolol has been extensively studied and is useful for control of hypertension perioperatively.

Calcium channel blockers are of little use for the acute management of hypertension, although sublingual administration of nifedipine is well recognised in the recovery period. Long-term blood pressure control is more appropriate with these drugs. The use of nimodipine and nicardipine in patients with subarachnoid haemorrhage is discussed elsewhere.

KEY POINTS

- Opioids in low doses have little effect on CMR, CBF and ICP.
- Abrupt use of naloxone is detrimental.
- Non-depolarising muscle relaxants have little effect on cerebral physiology.
- Suxemethonium is not contraindicated in neuroanaesthesia.
- Vasodilator drugs increase CBV and ICP but not necessarily CBF.
- α- and β-blockers appear to have little or no effect on ICP/CBF.

FURTHER READING

Coles JP, Monteiro JN, Brazier P, et al. Propofol anesthesia for craniotomy: a double-blind comparison of remifentanil, alfentanil and fenatanyl. J Neurosurg Anesthesiol 2000; 12(1): 15–20

Dahl A, Russell D, Nyberg-Hansen R, et al. Effect of nitroglycerin on cerebral circulation measured by transcranial doppler and SPECT. Stroke 1989; 20: 1733

Muzzi DA, Black S, Losasso TJ, et al. Labetalol and esmolol in the control of hypertension after intracranial surgery. Anesth Analg 1990; 70: 68

11

ANTICONVULSANTS

J. Monteiro

INTRODUCTION

The term *seizure* refers to a transient alteration in behaviour due to disorganised synchronous and rhythmic firing of populations of neurones. *Epilepsy* refers to a disorder of brain function characterised by the periodic and unpredictable occurrence of seizures. Seizure classification and treatments are shown in Table 11.1.

MECHANISMS OF ANTICONVULSANT ACTION

The mechanisms of action of anticonvulsants can be divided into three major categories:

1. *Action on sodium channels* Carbamazepine, phenytoin, lamotrigine and valproate all limit sustained repetitive neuronal firing by prolonging the inactivation of sodium ion channels. This reduces the ability of neurones to fire at high frequencies. The inactivated channel itself remains open but is blocked by the inactivation gate.
2. *Action on GABAergic neurones*
   a. Reduced GABA metabolism: Valproate, vigabatrim and gabapentin all inhibit the enzyme GABA transaminase responsible for GABA metabolism. Increased levels of available GABA result in hyperpolarisation of neurones.

   b. Increased GABA response: Benzodiazepines and barbiturates act at the GABA receptor to enhance chloride ion influx in response to GABA and produce a hyperpolarisation of the nerve membrane.
3. *Calcium channel blockade*: Valproate, ethosuximide and dimethadione reduce calcium ion flow through T type calcium ion channels and reduce the pacemaker current known as the T current.

DOSING SCHEDULES AND SIDE-EFFECTS

Usual daily doses and therapeutic serum concentrations are shown in Table 11.2. Side-effect profiles of the more common anticonvulsants are shown in Table 11.3. Dose regimes used in the management of status epilepticus are outlined in Chapter 46. Ventilatory support is usually required in status and drug dose can be titrated to desired effect on EEG.

COMBINATION THERAPY AND INTERACTIONS

Combinations of anticonvulsants are sometimes used on the basis that therapeutic effects are additive while individual toxicity is reduced. Toxicity, however, may be enhanced with combination therapy. A second drug

Table 11.1 Classification of seizures and treatment		
Seizure type	Usual anticonvulsant	Alternative treatment
A. Partial seizures (confined to local areas of brain):		
1. Simple partial (no alteration to consciousness)	Carbamazepine, phenytoin, phenobarbitone	Gabapentin, lamotrigine
2. Complex partial (altered consciousness)	As above	
3. Partial with secondarily generalised tonic clonic seizures	Carbamazepine, phenytoin	Primidone, valproate
B. Generalised seizures		
Absence seizure	Ethosuximide, valproate	Clonazepam, lamotrigine
Myoclonic atonic	Valproate	Clonazepam
Tonic clonic seizure (grand mal)	Phenytoin, carbamazepine, valproate	Phenobarbitone, primidone
Status epilepticus	Diazepam, phenytoin	Phenobarbitone, thiopentone

Table 11.2 Therapeutic serum levels and dosing schedules of common anticonvulsants

Drug	Dose in adults (mg)	Dose in children (mg/kg)	Therapeutic serum concentration (μg/ml)
Phenytoin	300–400	4–7	10–20
Carbamazepine	600–1200	20–30	6–12
Valproate	1000–3000	15–60	50–100
Clonazepam	1500–2000	0.01–0.2	0.013–0.072
Phenobarbitone	60–180	5–8	0.06–0.18

Table 11.3 Side-effect (S/E) profile of common anticonvulsants

Drug	Dose related S/E	Idiosyncratic S/E	Long term S/E
Phenytoin	Ataxia, tremor, nystagmus, lethargy, dystonia, confusion	Rashes, lymphadenopathy, blood dyscrasias, liver damage, SLE	Gingival hyperplasia, hirsuitism, neuropathy, folate deficiency, osteomalacia
Carbamazepine	Drowsiness, ataxia, diplopia, hyponatremia	Stevens-Johnson syndrome, Rashes, dyspepsia, blood dyscrasias, cholestatic jaundice, acute renal failure	Gynaecomastia, galactorrhoea, thromboembolism, impotence, aggression
Valproate	Nausea, anorexia, tremors, ataxia, drowsiness	Rashes, sedation, alopecia, hepatic necrosis, thrombocytopenia	Hearing loss, vasculitis, menstrual irregularities, weight gain
Phenobarbitone	Drowsiness, nystagmus, ataxia	Rashes, SLE, paradoxical excitement	Folate deficiency, neuropathy, osteomalacia

should be added to the dosing regime only if seizures persist despite therapeutic serum drug levels or intolerable side-effects of the first-line drug. Interactions between anticonvulsants are complex, highly variable and unpredictable and may enhance toxicity without corresponding increases in anti-epileptic effect. The mechanism of interaction is usually due to hepatic microsomal enzyme induction or inhibition. Displacement of drugs from protein binding sites is usually not a contributory factor. Monitoring of serum drug levels is therefore mandatory with combination therapy.

FURTHER READING

Commission on the classification and terminology of the International league against epilepsy. Proposal for revised classification of epilepsies and epileptic syndromes. Epilepsia 1989; 30: 389–399

McDonald RL, Kelly KM. Antiepileptic drug mechanisms of action Epilepsia 1993; 34 (supplement 5): S1–S8

McNamara JO. Drugs effective in the management of epilepsies. In: Molinoff PB, Ruddon RW, Gilman AG (eds) Goodman and Gilman's The pharmacological basis of therapeutics, 9th Edn. New York: McGraw Hill, 1996; pp. 461–486

Section 4
NEUROANAESTHESIA

12

CRANIOTOMY FOR SPACE OCCUPYING LESIONS

C. Duffy

CLASSIFICATION

Space occupying lesions comprise tumours, vascular lesions (Chapter 13), abscesses and haematomas (spontaneous or traumatic). Presenting symptoms are commonly those of raised ICP, seizures or neurological deficit.

TUMOURS

Primary Lesions

Most primary lesions (55–60%) are supratentorial. *Gliomas* are the most common primary brain tumour and range from relatively benign pilocytic and well-differentiated astrocytomas to aggressive anaplastic astrocytomas and glioblastoma multiforme. On CT or MRI, malignant lesions have a contrast-enhancing rim with surrounding oedema. Gliomas are treated with varying combinations of chemotherapy, radio-therapy and surgery.

Meningiomas are extraparenchymal lesions and may be very vascular. The surgical goal is complete excision. *Colloid cysts of third ventricle* usually present with obstructive hydrocephalus.

Secondary Lesions

These comprise 40–45% of supratentorial tumours arising mostly from the lung (50%) and breast (10%). Excision of solitary lesions is justified in those whose underlying disease is well controlled. *Abscesses* may extend from local sinus or ear infections especially in immunocompromised patients, or are blood-borne in those with right-to-left cardiac shunts and intravenous drug abusers.

PREOPERATIVE MANAGEMENT

Specific preoperative information to obtain includes an accurate assessment of the acute neurological condition together with preoperative Glasgow coma scale (GCS), an examination of radiological images and an evaluation of concurrent disease (e.g. underlying chronic respiratory disease in those with lung metastases). Preoperative examination of CT and/or MRI scan provides information about lesion size, ease of surgical access, positioning of the patient and indirect information regarding likelihood of blood loss and ICP, remembering that patients may have raised ICP even if not evident clinically on CT or MRI.

Premedication is only given if the patient is particularly anxious, provided there is no evidence of raised ICP. In this case, consider a short-acting benzodiazepine. Medications such as anticonvulsants and steroids are continued in the perioperative period. Steroids may reduce oedema and improve symptoms in patients with malignant lesions and abscesses.

INTRAOPERATIVE MANAGEMENT

The aims of anaesthetic management are:

1. Smooth induction.
2. Haemodynamic stability (hypotension can lead to ischaemia in areas of impaired autoregulation; hypertension increases the risk of haemorrhage and vasogenic oedema).
3. Relaxed brain (for optimal surgical access, decreasing the risks of retractor injury).
4. Cerebral protection if required.
5. Rapid and smooth emergence.

Induction

Invasive blood pressure monitoring may be established prior to induction. Induction is performed using an intravenous anaesthetic agent of choice (Chapter 8), together with a non-depolarising muscle relaxant and an opiate (fentanyl, alfentanil, sufentanil and remifentanil have all been used successfully). Normotension should be maintained by anticipating stimuli and preventing haemodynamic responses. The hypertensive response to laryngoscopy and intubation can be obtunded with an additional bolus of intravenous induction agent, a short-acting opioid β-blocker or intravenous lidocaine.

After induction, a nasopharyngeal temperature probe and urinary catheter should be inserted. A central venous line should be inserted if there is an indication (e.g. cardiorespiratory disease, anticipated blood loss). A pulmonary artery catheter may be further required in severe cardiac disease. Further neuromonitoring, e.g. EEG, somatosensory evoked potentials (SSEPs) and jugular bulb catheter ($SjvO_2$) can also be established if required.

Insertion of skull-pin head-holder is a potent stimulus and the hypertensive response should be pre-empted either by local anaesthetic infiltration, an additional dose of induction agent or a supplemental dose of opiate. A CSF drainage device may also be inserted prior to surgery.

Maintenance

The patient's head should be positioned so that venous drainage is not obstructed. The choice of anaesthetic drugs is largely at the discretion of the anaesthetist. Total intravenous anaesthesia (using propofol) and/or inhalational agents (using isoflurane or sevoflurane) can be used. Most anaesthetists choose a technique allowing for control of ICP and rapid emergence at the completion of surgery. The lungs are ventilated aiming for a $PaCO_2$ between 4.0 and 4.5kPa. Mannitol 0.5–1 g/kg is given approximately 30–60 minutes prior to dura opening. Many anaesthetists allow body temperature to drift to 34–36°C, although there is no good evidence that this is beneficial. Rewarming is commenced as soon as the dura is closed. One of the intraoperative complications is acute cerebral oedema, the management of which is given in Table 12.1.

Fluid management

CVP is used as a guide to maintain normovolaemia. Dextrose-containing fluids should be avoided, as there is an increased incidence of neurological deficit associated with hyperglycaemia and focal cerebral oedema in experimental models. Blood products should be available in the event of major bleeding aiming for resuscitation to a haematocrit of 0.30. Thromboplastin release causing disseminated intravascular coagulation (DIC) may occur and appropriate clotting factors should be given early.

Table 12.1 Management of intraoperative cerebral oedema

- *Optimise ventilation and blood gases*
- *Maximise venous drainage*
- *Deepen anaesthesia:* bolus intravenous anaesthetic agent, adjust inhalational agent concentration
- *Diuretics:* Mannitol (0.25–1.0 g/kg) ± furosemide (0.25–0.5 mg/kg)
- *CSF drainage*
- *Minimise $CMRO_2$:* bolus lidocaine; thiopentone or propofol infusion
- *Consider further doses of diuretic and CSF drainage.*

POSTOPERATIVE MANAGEMENT

Patients with a depressed level of consciousness preoperatively usually require postoperative ventilation and monitoring in intensive care, otherwise, provided the intraoperative course is uneventful, patients with a preoperative GCS of 13–15 can be extubated once they open eyes to command and have demonstrated a gag reflex. The overall aim is to achieve a smooth emergence with minimal coughing and straining which may be reduced by intravenous lidocaine (1.5 mg/kg) a few minutes prior to extubation. Hypertension at this stage can be treated with a bolus of β-blocker (esmolol 0.5 mg/kg or labetalol 10–20 mg). Direct vasodilators may increase CBF and ICP and should be avoided. In patients with delayed emergence in whom a drug or metabolic cause has been excluded, a neurosurgical complication should be suspected and an immediate CT scan should be arranged.

After routine craniotomy, analgesic requirements are usually satisfied by mild opiates such as codeine phosphate or non-steroidal analgesics (if not contraindicated). Potent opiates are often not required and may cause some degree of respiratory depression.

KEY POINTS

- Preoperatively assess neurological state, determine the presence of raised ICP and optimise underlying disease.
- A total intravenous and/or inhalational anaesthesia technique may be used.
- Maintain normotension, normovolaemia and a relaxed brain intraoperatively.
- Aim for smooth, rapid emergence postoperatively.
- Potent postoperative opioid analgesics are usually not required. Avoid sedative drugs.

FURTHER READING

McDonald JD, Rosenblum ML. Gliomas. In: Rengachary SS, Wilkins RH (eds) Principles of neurosurgery. London: Wolfe 1994; 26.2–26.32

Todd MM, Warner DS. Neuroanesthesia: a critical review. In: Rogers MC, Tinker JH, Covino BG, Longnecker DE (eds) Principles and practice of anesthesiology. St Louis: Mosby-Year Book 1993, pp. 1599–1648

13

CRANIOTOMY FOR VASCULAR LESIONS

C. Duffy

CEREBRAL ANEURYSM

A cerebral aneurysm is a diverticulum arising from vessels of the circle of Willis, usually at a bifurcation. They occur in 2–5% of the population and are three times as common in females as males. Over 90% of all aneurysms involve the anterior circulation and about 10% involve the posterior circulation (see Chapter 2).

PREDISPOSING FACTORS

Aneurysm formation is predisposed in hypertension, pregnancy and a number of genetic and collagen abnormalities including those with a family history of cerebral aneurysm, coarctation of the aorta, fibromuscular dysplasia, polycystic kidney disease and type III collagen deficiency.

CLASSIFICATION

Aneurysms are classified as small (< 12 mm diameter – 78% of all aneurysms); large (12–24 mm – 20% of aneurysms) or giant (> 24 mm – 2% of aneurysms) and most present as a haemorrhage into the subarachnoid space (SAH).

NATURAL HISTORY

The risk of rupture is estimated at 0.05–6%. Factors associated with an increased risk of rupture include: larger sized aneurysms, previous SAH, aneurysm location (especially basilar tip aneurysms) and increased patient age. Rupture occurs more frequently in the 40 to 60-year age group. When rupture occurs, it is related to hypertensive episodes. In the event of SAH, one-third of patients do not reach hospital, one-third have a poor outcome and one-third are functional survivors. The risk of perioperative mortality increases with worsening neurological grade at presentation (see below).

PRESENTATION

Subarachnoid Haemorrhage

Headache is the presenting symptom in 85–95% of patients. Other symptoms are brief loss of consciousness, nausea, vomiting, photophobia or neurological deficits (see Tables 13.1 and 13.2). Bleeding increases ICP and leads to reduced CPP. The subsequent reduction in CBF stops bleeding. If CBF recovers, reactive hyperaemia allows function to improve. Non-survivors are those in whom CBF does not recover.

Table 13.1 Hunt and Hess classification of intracranial aneurysms

Category	Criteria
0	Unruptured aneurysm
I	Asymptomatic or minimal headache and slight nuchal rigidity
II	Moderate to severe headache, nuchal rigidity, ± cranial nerve palsy
III	Drowsiness, confusion, or mild focal deficit
IV	Stupor, moderate to severe hemiparesis, possibly early decerebrate rigidity and vegetative disturbances
V	Deep coma, decerebrate rigidity, moribund appearance

Hydrocephalus

This may occur if blood enters the ventricles and obstructs the flow of CSF. Absence of CSF flow is associated with vasospasm (see below) and a further disruption of the blood–brain barrier.

Re-bleeding

Thirty per cent of ruptured cerebral aneurysms rebleed within 2 weeks with half of these occurring within the first 24 hours.

Cardiac Dysfunction

This is frequently associated with SAH and probably mediated by a variety of mechanisms including catecholamine release triggered by SAH, direct trauma to cerebral autonomic control mechanisms and a hypothalamic neurogenic mechanism. This may lead to hypertension, dysrhythmias (especially ventricular ectopics that may progress to life-threatening ventricular dysrhythmias) and pulmonary oedema.

Table 13.2 World Federation of Neurological Surgeons (WFNS) SAH Scale

WFNS grade	GCS score	Motor deficit
I	15	Absent
II	14–13	Absent
III	14–13	Present
IV	12–7	Present or absent
V	6–3	Present or absent

Ventricular wall function is depressed in 30% of patients. A diffuse myocardial ischaemia occurs in 50% of patients with widespread ST segment and T wave changes on ECG. The ECG abnormalities probably reflect the severity of neurologic dysfunction.

Vasospasm

This occurs in 30–40% of patients admitted to hospital, typically 4–9 days post-SAH. It rarely occurs within the first 3 days, peaks in 7–10 days and resolves over 10–14 days. The diagnosis rests on clinical signs of a new neurological deficit and decreased level of consciousness. Other causes need to be excluded such as re-bleed, hydrocephalus, seizures, oedema, electrolyte abnormalities, drug effects and other medical complications. Angiography is the 'gold standard' investigation to confirm diagnosis and may be abnormal even in the absence of clinical evidence of vasospasm. Vasospasm can also be suggested by trends in transcranial Doppler ultrasonography of cerebral blood flow velocity . The cause of vasospasm is uncertain, however the amount of subarachnoid blood correlates with its occurrence and severity, as does the degree of abnormality in CBF autoregulation and CO_2 reactivity. The microscopic appearance is suggestive of a vasculopathy triggered by inflammatory mediators released from blood and its breakdown products. These include oxyhaemoglobin, bilirubin, endothelin and superoxide radicals, which in turn affect nitric oxide production, calcium release and prostaglandin synthesis. All of these cause vasoconstriction of cerebral arteries. The occurrence of vasospasm doubles the risk of mortality. Nimodipine has been shown to improve outcome for SAH despite not preventing vasospasm. It should be started on admission with an oral or nasogastric dose of 60 mg every 4 hours, or a reduced intravenous dose if hypotension is a problem. The reason for improved outcome remains uncertain.

PREOPERATIVE MANAGEMENT

The patient's acute condition is assessed and graded according to Hunt and Hess (Table 13.1) or World Federation of Neurological Surgeons (Table 13.2) scales. With worsening grades, CBF autoregulation and CO_2 response also deteriorate. Grades I and II (Hunt and Hess scale) often have near normal ICP values.

Cardiac function must be assessed and optimised. Serious dysrhythmias need to be treated. Fluid resuscitation with invasive monitoring may be required preoperatively especially in poor grade patients as they are often intravascularly depleted. Hypovolaemia should be avoided to help prevent further ischaemia in areas of vasospasm. Hyponatraemia may be present from either a true SIADH or a central salt wasting syndrome. Previous medical history should be noted. Avoid premedication unless the patient has grade I SAH and is particularly anxious. Nimodipine should be continued throughout the perioperative period. This is best administered through a central venous catheter.

Early surgery soon after aneurysm rupture reduces the risk of re-bleeding but does not affect the incidence of vasospasm. Early surgery is also technically difficult due to oedema but facilitates medical and neuroradiological treatment of vasospasm if it occurs later.

INTRAOPERATIVE MANAGEMENT

Monitoring

Direct arterial blood pressure, central venous pressure monitoring and a urinary catheter are mandatory. Pulmonary arterial pressure monitoring should be used if impaired myocardial function is suspected. More specialised intraoperative monitoring may include jugular bulb oximetry, transcranial Doppler, EEG or evoked potentials.

Induction

Aneurysmal rupture is related to transmural pressure across the wall of the aneurysm (MAP–ICP). Rupture occurs in 1–2% of anaesthetic inductions with a mortality rate approaching 75%. Hypertension increases the risk of aneurysm rupture as does aggressive hyperventilation and hypocapnia. In addition, hypotension can lead to ischaemia in areas of impaired autoregulation. Accordingly, the objective should be normotension during the induction and maintenance phases of anaesthesia and large changes in transmural pressure should be avoided. Invasive blood pressure monitoring should commence prior to induction and supplemental doses of induction agent or high dose opiate may be required to avoid pressor responses of laryngoscopy and intubation.

Maintenance

A technique allowing for titration of blood pressure is important. A propofol infusion and/or inhalational technique are acceptable. Mannitol and mild hyperventilation after dura opening may be required to reduce brain swelling permitting better exposure.

Temporary Clipping/Induced Hypotension

During dissection, the surgeon may reduce tension in the aneurysm using a temporary clip on a feeding vessel or the anaesthetist may induce systemic hypotension using short–acting vasodilators or β–blockers. The minimum MAP to prevent ischaemia has never been established.

Temporary clips are applied more frequently and the risk of ischaemia is high if occlusion is prolonged (> 10–15 minutes). Ideally, electrophysiological monitoring should be used as a guide to the safe duration of temporary clipping. Use of pharmacological neuroprotection, e.g. bolus doses of intravenous anaesthetic agents together with hypothermia may allow the safe duration of temporary clipping to be extended but controlled trials are lacking. Induced *hypertension* at this time may help improve collateral blood flow.

Following *permanent* clip application, cerebral perfusion may be improved by allowing blood pressure to increase. This should be weighed against the potential for myocardial ischaemia. In the presence of known unclipped aneurysms, normotension should be continued.

MANAGEMENT OF INTRAOPERATIVE ANEURYSM RUPTURE

This may be suspected before aneurysm exposure by a Cushing's reflex with hypertension ± bradycardia and treatment is outlined in Table 13.3.

Controlled hypotension, to a MAP of 50 mmHg, is reserved for situations where intraoperative aneurysm rupture has occurred and the rate of blood loss needs to be slowed in order to achieve surgical control.

POSTOPERATIVE MANAGEMENT

A fast, smooth emergence enables early clinical assessment and a diagnostic CT or angiogram should be performed if the neurological assessment is not satisfactory. Blood pressure should be closely monitored

and controlled pharmacologically if required. Hypertension is frequently seen as a response to restore CPP and CBF. Systolic pressures over 240 mmHg (MAP > 150 mmHg) can lead to vasogenic oedema.

ARTERIOVENOUS MALFORMATIONS

An arteriovenous malformation (AVM) is a congenital intraparenchymal cluster of arterial-venous communications. Over 70–90% are supratentorial and 10% are infratentorial with 10–15% involving the dura. They present usually at age 20–40 years. Untreated, the risk of haemorrhage is 1–3% per year and the annual rate of death and disability is 4%.

The majority of patients (50–75%) present with intracerebral haemorrhage (ICH). Unlike aneurysms, haemorrhage is not related to hypertension and is usually venous in origin. Vasospasm and acute re-bleeding tend not to occur.

Other presenting symptoms include seizures, migraine-like headaches and a steal syndrome manifesting as a progressive neurological deficit.

Surgical risk of AVM excision is graded according to size, anatomy of feeding arteries and venous drainage, and location and eloquence of adjacent brain areas. Other therapeutic options are considered if surgical risk is high, i.e. endovascular embolisation or radiosurgery.

PATHOPHYSIOLOGY

AVMs are high-flow, low-resistance shunts and, if large, may steal normal perfusion from the surrounding brain. Up to 10% are associated with aneurysms, which probably develop because of increased flow through the AVM. These often resolve following AVM resection.

Table 13.3 Treatment guidelines for ruptured intraoperative aneurysm

100% inspired O₂

Fluid resuscitation

Controlled hypotension:	MAP of 50 mmHg reduces the rate of blood loss aiding surgical control. MAP is normalised after bleeding is controlled.
Neuroprotection strategies:	Boluses of thiopentone, etomidate or propofol to produce burst suppression or an isoelectric EEG; Mild hypothermia (35–36°C); Mannitol (0.25–1 g/kg) if significant brain swelling; For prolonged temporary clipping or uncontrolled bleeding: cool to 33°C and commence infusions of thiopentone (1 g/h) or propofol (100–200 mg/h)

PREOPERATIVE MANAGEMENT

The presence of cerebral aneurysms should be noted.

INTRAOPERATIVE MANAGEMENT

Bleeding from AVMs can be large, rapid and sustained. Blood products must be readily available. As haemorrhage is usually venous in origin, avoid increases in jugular venous pressure that can be transmitted to the cerebral circulation (i.e. care with internal jugular lines, ETT fixation tapes, avoiding head down, PEEP). Management of acute brain swelling intraoperatively is described in Chapter 12.

Deliberate hypotension may assist the surgeon in the visualisation and ligation of arterial feeders. However, it carries the risk of causing ischaemia in non-autoregulating surrounding brain and may lead to venous thrombosis. A decision about blood pressure management should be made on an individual basis after discussion with the surgical team.

POSTOPERATIVE MANAGEMENT AND COMPLICATIONS

Hyperaemia producing oedema or haemorrhage and intracranial hypertension may occur in the postoperative period due to:

1. 'Normal perfusion pressure breakthrough' (NPPB) where hypoperfused brain surrounding the AVM theoretically loses the ability to autoregulate and restoration of normal CBF after the AVM is removed leads to microhaemorrhages and diffuse swelling. Staged removal by excision or embolisation should theoretically allow the surrounding brain to regain autoregulatory mechanisms.
2. Postoperative haemorrhage from residual AVM.
3. 'Occlusive hyperaemia' where venous outflow obstruction predisposes to haemorrhage if arterial feeders are not completely occluded. It is also possible that venous obstruction may result in hypoperfusion due to stagnation of CBF.

Hyperaemia is a major source of postoperative morbidity/mortality.

The risk of seizures following AVM resection approaches 50%. If the intraoperative course has been uneventful, the patient should be extubated at the end of the procedure. Because of the risk of hyperaemia, it is important to avoid hypertension at the time of emergence. The use of β-blockers may reduce blood pressure without delaying emergence.

If intraoperative bleeding has been excessive or there is evidence of brain swelling, the patient should be ventilated postoperatively with ICP monitoring. Blood pressure should be maintained in the low normal range. Continuation of muscle paralysis minimises the risk of venous congestion due to coughing and straining and other neuroprotective strategies should be considered (Chapter 40).

KEY POINTS

Aneurysms

- SAH is associated with cardiac dysfunction and fluid and electrolyte imbalance.
- Vasospasm and further bleeding are complications of aneurysm rupture.
- Avoid large changes in transmural pressure (MAP-ICP) across the wall of unclipped aneurysms.
- CPP should be optimal at the time of temporary clip application.
- Maintain normovolaemia if intraoperative rupture occurs.

AVMs

- Intraoperative blood loss can be rapid and large.
- Onset of cerebral oedema can be rapid and occur intraoperatively soon after AVM resection.
- Postoperative hyperaemia worsens outcome.
- Postoperative blood pressure should be maintained in the low normal range.

FURTHER READING

The International Study of Unruptured Intracranial Aneurysm investigators. Unruptured intracranial aneurysms – risk of rupture and risks of surgical intervention. N Engl J Med 1998; 339: 1725–1733

Spetzler RF, Martin NA. A proposed grading system for arteriovenous malformations. J Neurosurg 1986; 65: 476–483

Guy J, McGrath BJ, Borel CO, Friedman AH, Warner DS. Perioperative management of aneurysmal subarachnoid hemorrhage: part 1. Operative management (review article). Anesth Analg 1995; 81: 1060–1072

McGrath BJ, Guy J, Borel CO, Friedman AH, Warner DS. Perioperative management of aneurysmal subarachnoid hemorrhage: part 2. Postoperative management (review article). Anesth Analg 1995; 81: 1295–1302

Young WL, Kader A, Prohovnik I, et al. Pressure autoregulation is intact after arteriovenous malformation resection. Neurosurgery 1993; 32: 491–497

Al-Rodhan NRF, Sundt TM, Piepgras DG, Nichols DA, Rufenacht D, Stevens LN. Occlusive hyperemia: a theory for the hemodynamic complications following resection of intracerebral arteriovenous malformations. J Neurosurg 1993; 78: 167–175

14

POSTERIOR FOSSA SURGERY

C. Goldsack

INTRODUCTION

The posterior fossa contains the cerebellum and the brainstem. The major sensory and motor pathways between the cerebrum and the rest of the body run through the posterior fossa. The brainstem also contains the vital centres controlling cardiovascular and respiratory function. Failure of these centres is incompatible with life. The anatomy of the posterior fossa is given in Chapter 3.

PATHOLOGY

TUMOURS

Primary brain tumours such as gliomas and astrocytomas are the commonest indication for posterior fossa surgery. Malignant tumours from elsewhere can metastasise to the cerebellum. Benign tumours include meningiomas and also acoustic neuromas (Schwannomas), which arise from the VIIIth cranial nerve, often in the cerebellopontine angle. Haemangioblastomas can develop in the cerebellum and frequently secrete erythropoietin, resulting in polcythaemia.

VASCULAR LESIONS

These are uncommon in the posterior fossa. Aneurysms tend to occur on the posterior-inferior cerebellar artery (PICA) which is an important supply to the midbrain. Vasospasm will therefore have serious consequences. Small vessels impinging on cranial nerves in the posterior fossa can result in symptoms such as trigeminal neuralgia. Surgical decompression has a good success rate.

FORAMEN MAGNUM DECOMPRESSION

In the young this is usually for congenital abnormalities such as Arnold–Chiari malformation; in the elderly, degenerative changes can occur.

POSITIONING

PRONE POSITION

This position offers good access to midline structures but bleeding can obscure the surgical field. Head-up tilt is employed to reduce haemorrhage but this increases the risk of air embolism. The chest and iliac crests should be well supported to ensure free movement of the abdomen during respiration. Pressure on the iliac vessels should be avoided, reducing the risk of deep venous thrombosis and improving emptying of the epidural venous sinuses. The head is fixed in clamps in preference to a horseshoe in order to minimise pressure on the face and eyes.

LATERAL POSITION

This is suitable for approaches to lesions not in the midline, particularly the cerebellopontine angle. A variation called the 'park bench' position is often used; so-called because of the resemblance to a tramp sleeping on a bench in the park. A pad should be placed under the body in the axilla to minimise weight on the lower arm and shoulder. The pelvis should be fixed with supports in front and behind. The lower leg is flexed at the hip and knee. The upper leg is kept straight and slightly externally rotated to lock the knee with the foot on a firm support, which will prevent the patient sliding down the table if significant head-up tilt is used. A pillow is placed between the legs. The lower arm is flexed across the body and the upper arm is taped along the upper side of the body. The head is fixed in pins. Excessive flexion of the neck can obstruct the internal jugular veins. This can be avoided by ensuring a two- or three-finger breadth gap between chin and sternal notch.

SITTING POSITION

This was widely used for posterior fossa surgery in the past. It provides good surgical access to midline structures, improves surgical orientation and allows good drainage of blood and CSF. However, there are increased risks of cord compression, pneumocephalus and venous air embolism. Hypotensive techniques increase the risks of ischaemic damage. Many authorities now contend that with modern anaesthetic techniques there is no place for the sitting position in neuroanaesthesia. However, excessive head-up tilt in other positions exposes the patient to similar risks.

ANAESTHETIC TECHNIQUE

The choice of particular agents is not critical but stable anaesthesia is paramount. The effects of a particular drug on blood pressure and neurophysiological monitoring should be considered. Muscle relaxation is best provided by continuous infusion (e.g. atracurium). This helps ventilation and prevents movement in a relatively lightly anaesthetised patient. If motor nerve function is monitored, such as the facial nerve during acoustic neuroma surgery, muscle relaxation must be discontinued and sufficient depth of anaesthesia must be provided. A remifentanil infusion is ideal in this situation.

A central venous line is usually required and access to the internal jugular veins may be difficult. Subclavian, antecubital fossa or femoral long lines are alternatives. A nasogastric tube should be inserted if there is any risk of postoperative bulbar dysfunction.

Neurophysiological monitoring is used frequently. Auditory evoked potentials are used for detecting dissection near the brainstem, particularly during acoustic neuroma surgery. When somatosensory and motor evoked potentials are monitored, they can be suppressed during deep anaesthesia.

Deliberate hypotension should be employed with caution if significant head-up tilt is used and because surgery near the brainstem can induce further hypotension and bradycardia.

The anaesthetic technique and intraoperative management is otherwise similar to that required for supratentorial craniotomy (Chapter 12).

POSTOPERATIVE MANAGEMENT

Extubation at the end of surgery should not occur if significant brainstem or cranial nerve injury has occurred. This may manifest as repeated episodes of intraoperative haemodynamic instability. Pulmonary oedema may be precipitated by large venous air embolism or after surgery to the floor of the fourth ventricle. Respiratory failure can occur suddenly, even when awake. Air may remain within the cranium for 2 weeks postoperatively which may be relevant should return to theatre become necessary.

COMPLICATIONS

AIR EMBOLISM

See Chapter 15.

ARRHYTHMIAS

These are often due to manipulation of the brainstem. Bradycardia can occur when the periventricular grey matter and the reticular formation are stimulated. Most arrhythmias occur during surgery near the pons and the roots of nerves V, IX and X. Severe hypertension can result from stimulation of the trigeminal nerve.

AIRWAY PROBLEMS

Macroglossia and upper airway swelling can occur following prolonged surgery in the prone position. This is due to obstruction of venous and lymphatic drainage. Cranial nerve damage can also cause serious airway problems.

NEUROLOGICAL COMPLICATIONS

Extreme neck flexion can cause midcervical quadraplegia. Prolonged surgery and hypotension are contributory factors. Surgery near the roots of nerves VII–X may lead to loss of airway reflexes, dysphagia and dysphonia. Peripheral nerve damage can result from faulty positioning. The brachial plexus, ulnar nerve and common peroneal nerve are most vulnerable.

PNEUMOCEPHALUS

Following a craniotomy, an air-filled space between the dura and arachnoid remains after CSF has leaked away during surgery and brain bulk is reduced. In the recovery period brain bulk increases again as cerebral oedema develops, arterial carbon dioxide concentrations increase and CSF reaccumulates. The trapped air then comes under increasing pressure. N_2O will worsen the situation. Pneumocephalus presents as delayed recovery or deteriorating neurological state and should always be considered if this occurs. Pneumocephalus can be reduced by discontinuing nitrous oxide 15 minutes before surgery finishes and by allowing the $PaCO_2$ to rise towards the end of the operation.

KEY POINTS

- The conduct of anaesthesia is similar to supratentorial surgery.
- The facial and peripheral nerves can be injured in the prone and lateral position.
- The sitting position has risks of venous air embolism and cerebral ischaemia.
- Haemodynamic instability occurs if the brainstem is manipulated.
- Extubation should be delayed if there are concerns of brainstem or cranial nerve injury.

FURTHER READING

Black S, Ockert DB, Oliver WC, et al. Outcome following posterior fossa craniectomy in the sitting or the horizontal positions. Anesthesiology 1988; 69: 49

McAlpine FS, Seckel BR. Complications of positioning. The peripheral nervous system. In: Martin TJ (ed.) Positioning in anesthesia and surgery. Philadelphia: WB Saunders, 1987

Marshall WK, Bedford RF, Miller ED. Cardiovascular responses in the seated position–impact of four anesthetic techniques. Anesth Analg 1983; 62: 648

Matjasko J, Petrozza P, Cohen M, et al. Anesthesia and surgery in the seated position: analysis of 554 cases. Neurosurgery 1985; 17: 695

15

AIR EMBOLISM

C. Goldsack

INTRODUCTION

A vein cut during surgery will normally collapse, which prevents air being sucked into the circulation. In posterior fossa surgery cut veins may not collapse: veins in the skull are held open by the surrounding bone, suboccipital veins are held open by cervical fascia, and the large venous sinuses are held open by the dura. Air can thus readily enter the circulation if these veins are opened. The incidence of air embolism is usually reported at between 25 and 40%. However, recent use of transoesophageal echocardiography has reported an incidence as high as 75%. In most cases the amount of air entering the circulation is small and may have little clinical importance.

PATHOPHYSIOLOGY

Air enters the venous system if the cut vein is positioned significantly above the level of the heart. It enters the right side of the heart and reduces cardiac output leading to systemic hypotension. Air also passes into the pulmonary arterial circulation, leading to a rise in pulmonary vascular resistance and an increase in pulmonary artery pressure. The ECG show signs of right ventricular strain and right ventricular failure may occur. Physiological dead space increases as air blocks the pulmonary circulation with many alveoli ventilated but not perfused. This in turn leads to a decrease in carbon dioxide excretion and a fall in end-tidal carbon dioxide tension. Central venous pressure (CVP) will rise as a result of obstruction to right ventricular outflow. This increase in CVP together with arrhythmias and the classical mill-wheel murmur on auscultation, however, are late signs.

If the patient has a patent foramen ovale there is potential for air to pass from the right atrium to the left atrium and thus into the systemic arterial circulation. This leads to emboli in any organ but has most serious consequences in the cerebral and coronary arteries.

DETECTION OF AIR EMBOLISM

Precordial Doppler Device

The altered reflection of ultrasonic beams from an air–gas interface means that precordial Doppler probes can detect bubbles of air in the circulation and can indicate air emboli as small as 1 ml; some critics claim that the device is oversensitive. An experienced observer is required. Diathermy machines will interfere with probe function.

Capnography

A continuous capnograph will show a fall in end-tidal carbon dioxide concentration as air enters the pulmonary circulation. It is less sensitive than the Doppler but is much easier to use. However, other causes of a fall in end-tidal carbon dioxide tensions, such as reduced cardiac output can cause confusion.

End-tidal Nitrogen

When air enters the pulmonary circulation there is a rise in end-tidal nitrogen, which mirrors the decrease in end-tidal carbon dioxide. However, nitrogen increase is more specific than end-tidal carbon dioxide and is not influenced by other cardiovascular changes.

Pulmonary Artery Pressure

Air embolism will increase the pulmonary artery pressure proportionally to the size of the embolism.

Pulse Oximetry

Oximetry will detect air embolism in the way that capnography does but it is an indicator of the magnitude of circulatory disturbance and provides an index of the progress of treatment.

Transoesophageal Echocardiography

A highly sensitive method of detecting intracardiac air and of diagnosing atrial septal defects.

PREVENTION OF AIR EMBOLISM

If N_2O is used during anaesthesia when an air embolism occurs, then N_2O will diffuse into the embolic bubbles and increase their size. If there is a significant air embolism, N_2O should be discontinued.

Volume loading patients to raise their CVPs will reduce the hydrostatic pressure gradient and reduce the likelihood of air embolism. Similarly, raising end-expiratory pressure may reduce the negative pressure in an open vein in the posterior fossa. However, PEEP will reduce venous return and may cause systemic hypotension.

Anti-gravity suits and medical anti-shock trousers help to reduce venous pooling in the lower limbs. The increase in venous pressure reduces postural hypotension and decreases the negative hydrostatic pressure in the posterior fossa.

A central venous catheter is a useful cardiovascular monitor and is a helpful diagnostic tool if air enters the circulation. It also provides a useful method of attempting to aspirate air from the right atrium.

MANAGEMENT OF AIR EMBOLISM

- Flood the operative field with saline and cover the wound with wet swabs to prevent further air entrainment.
- Ventilate with 100% oxygen, discontinue N_2O.
- Raise the venous pressure at the operative site, which can be done by squeezing the veins in the neck.
- Aspirate from the CVP catheter to try to aspirate air from the right atrium.
- If cardiovascular collapse occurs, standard resuscitative measures should be employed.

KEY POINTS

- Venous air embolism is more common with open skull veins, particularly in the posterior fossa.
- Intravascular air increases cardiac work and reduces cardiac output and gas exchange.
- Reducing hydrostatic pressure differences in open veins helps prevent air entry.

FURTHER READING

Cucchiara RF, Black S, Steinkeler JA. Anaesthesia for intracranial procedures. In: Barash P, Cullen B, Stoelting R (eds) Clinical anesthesia. Philadelphia: JB Lippincott, 1989, p. 849

Young ML, Smith DS, Murtagh F, et al. Comparison of surgical and anesthetic complications in neurosurgical patients experiencing venous air embolism in the sitting position. Neurosurgery 1986; 18: 157

16

ANAESTHESIA FOR ACOUSTIC NEUROMAS

A. Swami

INTRODUCTION

The term cerebellopontine angle (CPA) normally means the space bounded anteromedially by the lower pons and medulla; posteromedially by the cerebellum; and laterally by the petrous portion of the temporal bone. An acoustic neuroma is a schwannoma arising from the vestibular portion of CN VIII, occurring in the fifth and sixth decade of life with equal sex distribution, and account for about 80% of all CPA tumours. The primary presenting symptom is of hearing loss, but hemifacial spasm and tic douloureux can also rarely occur. Hydrocephalus occurs with large tumours.

Acoustic neuroma classification, treatment and mortality are according to tumour size measured on MRI:

SIZE		MORTALITY
• Small	0–15 mm	0%
• Medium	16–30 mm	< 1%
• Large	> 31 mm	4–7%

The main concern in surgery for small tumours is preservation of CN VII and hearing function. Facial paralysis is arguably the most disturbing and devastating complication.

For large tumours, the aim is to protect the brainstem and lower cranial nerves including CN VII.

SURGICAL APPROACHES

The *suboccipital* approach can be universally applied regardless of size and gives excellent exposure. Although there is a possibility of cerebellar retraction, this approach allows a good probability of hearing preservation and a low incidence of anterior inferior cerebellar artery occlusion.

With the *translabyrinthine* approach, exposure of the tumour is accomplished at the expense of bone removal rather than cerebellar or brainstem retraction and allows early identification of CN VII. However, hearing is necessarily destroyed.

The *middle fossa* approach is successful for small tumours especially when hearing preservation is a goal although is technically difficult due to lack of anatomical landmarks.

PREOPERATIVE CONSIDERATIONS

Although these tumours generally do not invade tissues but tend to displace them, larger tumours cause symptoms and signs of brainstem distortion. Hydrocephalus may be present and requires treatment before definitive tumour surgery. The preoperative evalua-

tion is otherwise similar to that of posterior fossa lesions (see Chapter 14). Premedication should be reserved for those with small tumours and who are neurologically intact.

INTRAOPERATIVE CONSIDERATIONS

Although these operations are usually prolonged, a smooth rapid wake up is still required to allow for neurological assessment. For patients with large tumours, total intravenous anaesthesia (TIVA) is preferred and inhalational agents avoided. This can be achieved using a propofol infusion and should be supplemented by an opiate. Fentanyl, Alfentanil and Remifentanil have all been used for this purpose. As facial nerve monitoring is used during the procedure, further non-depolarising muscle relaxants after intubation should be avoided. Care should therefore be taken to maintain a sufficient depth of anaesthesia to avoid movement intraoperatively. Maintenance of temperature and fluid balance is essential and both of these should be carefully monitored. Mild hypothermia (35°C) is frequently employed.

Positioning of the patient may be lateral, or more frequently the supine position. Care should be taken in the supine lateral position as obstruction of jugular vein can occur if the head is excessively rotated.

Surgical manipulation of brainstem structures may cause cardiovascular instability, and this should be reported to the surgeon. These responses should be preserved and anticholinergic or long-acting beta-blocking drugs should be avoided where possible.

Monitoring

In addition to the routine monitoring used for a posterior fossa operation, specific monitoring is also employed. Facial nerve monitoring is routinely used which consists of a stimulator and tremogram to detect facial muscle movement via a speaker. Auditory brainstem response recording can be used in patients with serviceable hearing.

Emergence

With large tumour resection, elective postoperative ventilation with paralysis in an ICU environment may be required. This facilitates control of blood pressure and prevents coughing or straining thereby reducing the possibility of haematoma formation in the operative site. Furthermore, difficult dissection of a large tumour will cause oedema of the brainstem and/or lower cranial nerves. This will obtund the cough or swallow reflex, which may delay extubation.

POSTOPERATIVE COMPLICATIONS

In addition to the complications that occur for any posterior fossa operation, additional complications for acoustic neuroma surgery include:

* hydrocephalus 1–2%
* CSF leak 6–14%
* meningitis 1–5%
* haematoma 0–6%
* CN VII paralysis 0–18%.

KEY POINTS

* Acoustic neuromas arise from CN VIII

* Anaesthetic implications are similar to those for posterior fossa surgery
* Facial nerve monitoring requires the patient to be unparalysed
* Surgery is often prolonged
* Cardiovascular instability may occur intraoperatively
* Airway reflexes may be obtunded particularly with large tumours.

FURTHER READING

Sterkers JM, Charachon R, Sterkers O (eds). Acoustic neuroma and skull base surgery. Kugler Publications, Amsterdam 1995, pp. 137–163, 439–442

17

EPILEPSY SURGERY

M. Smith

INTRODUCTION

Epilepsy occurs in approximately 1 in 200 of the population. It is a chronic illness due to an underlying disorder of neuronal activity, which is characterised by recurrent seizure activity. Despite considerable progress in the medical management of epilepsy and the development of new anti-convulsants, some patients remain refractory to therapy or develop intolerable side-effects. Surgery is an alternative and increasingly favourable option for patients with a discrete seizure focus.

PATHOPHYSIOLOGY

Epilepsy may be longstanding or develop de novo secondary to another pathology (e.g. brain tumour). Under normal circumstances electrical activity is well controlled within the brain, but in epileptic patients regulatory functions are altered. A group of neurones develop the capacity to produce spontaneous burst discharges which are recognised as inter-ictal spikes on the EEG. Failure of normal inhibitory processes allows spread of these discharges to surrounding areas, resulting in uncontrolled neuronal firing and seizure activity. Changes in membrane flux, impaired GABA-mediated synaptic inhibition and alterations in local neurotransmitter levels are implicated in this process.

The epilepsies may usefully be classified into generalised and partial types (Table 17.1). Generalised seizures involve both hemispheres and are characterised by an initial loss of consciousness. Partial epilepsies occur when the initial discharge is limited to one area of the brain. Simple partial seizures are caused by a localised discharge and there is no impairment of consciousness. In complex partial seizures the initial focal discharge spreads widely and secondary loss of consciousness occurs. This is the most common seizure disorder and includes temporal lobe epilepsy. High quality MRI has demonstrated that a high proportion of such patients has hippocampal sclerosis, and extended temporal lobectomy may offer a reduction of seizure frequency and severity.

ANTICONVULSANT THERAPY

Choice of anticonvulsant medication is determined by seizure type, seizure history, age of the patient and side-effects. Monotherapy is sufficient to control seizures in many patients but some require addition of second- or third-line agents (see Chapter 11).

PREOPERATIVE ASSESSMENT

The pattern, type and frequency of seizures should be noted. Co-existing medical problems are frequently encountered. Anticonvulsant levels should be measured and attention given to the potential side-effects of therapy. Drugs should be continued into the perioperative period and doses adjusted to ensure adequate plasma levels.

Premedication with a benzodiazepine is acceptable in most patients but should be avoided if intraoperative recording of inter-ictal spike activity is planned. A sympathetic visit from the anaesthetist reduces the need for pharmacological premedication under such circumstances.

INTRAOPERATIVE MANAGEMENT

Specific requirements for the management of a patient undergoing epilepsy surgery include the recording of intraoperative cerebral electrical activity and/or activation of the epileptic focus. Knowledge of the effects of anaesthetic agents on the EEG allows a rational choice of technique to be made (see Chapter 58).

Neurosurgery for medically intractable epilepsy may be carried out under general anaesthesia or with local anaesthesia and sedation. General anaesthesia is preferred in the UK but in patients in whom resection margins might impinge upon eloquent areas an awake procedure is preferable (see Chapter 18). In some patients, it is necessary to map EEG spike activity intraoperatively, to allow mapping of the epileptic focus and aid planning of the surgical resection margins. After dural opening, a small electrode grid is placed on the brain surface and allows the underlying cortical activity (the electrocorticogram – ECoG) to be recorded.

The anaesthetic techniques employed during epilepsy surgery are similar to those for any intracranial procedure with special attention given to the choice of

---

Table 17.1 Classification of the epilepsies

Generalised epilepsy
Generalised absence – petit mal
Generalised tonic-clonic – grand mal
Myoclonic
Tonic/atonic – drop attacks

Partial epilepsy
Complex partial – temporal lobe epilepsy
Simple partial

anaesthetic agent if intraoperative ECoG recording is indicated. Careful titration of end-tidal concentration of a volatile agent in combination with moderate doses of a short-acting opioid allows a depth of anaesthesia to be maintained which does not interfere with ECoG recording whilst minimising the risk of awareness. Alternatively, anaesthesia may be maintained by propofol infusion, although the effect on the ECoG is not yet fully characterised. Neuromuscular blockade should be maintained during the lighter stages of anaesthesia necessary for ECoG recording and monitoring of neuromuscular function is essential because of interactions between muscle relaxant and anticonvulsants. Blood pressure may be controlled by incremental opioid and labetolol infusion. In patients in whom intraoperative spike activity is not observed, it may be necessary for the anaesthetist to administer proconvulsant anaesthetic drugs. Small doses of methohexitone, thiopentone, propofol, fentanyl and alfentanil have all been successfully used for this purpose.

Intraoperative seizures during general anaesthesia are rare but may be masked by neuromuscular blockade. Unexpected tachycardia, hypertension or increases in end-tidal CO_2 are suspicious warning signs. ECoG can confirm the diagnosis. An intravenous bolus of propofol or thiopentone, followed by deepening of anaesthesia is usually sufficient to bring seizures under control.

POSTOPERATIVE CARE

The patient should be nursed in a neurosurgical intensive care/high dependency unit following surgery for epilepsy. Seizures may occur in the immediate postoperative period and if untreated may progress to status epilepticus. Seizures may be precipitated by metabolic changes, hypercarbia, drugs or by the underlying epilepsy (Table 17.2). A CT scan is helpful in excluding a 'surgical' cause of postoperative seizures. To avoid cerebral damage, seizures should be treated aggressively with benzodiazepines, thiopentone or propofol. Recurrent seizures may require top-up doses of long-acting anticonvulsant drugs or the introduction of adjuvant therapy (see Chapter 46).

Table 17.2 Factors which predispose to seizures

Anaesthetic factors
Proconvulsant anaesthetic agents (e.g. methohexitone, enflurane)
Light anaesthesia
Hypocarbia/hypercarbia
Hypoxaemia

Metabolic factors
Hypoglycaemia
Hyponatraemia/hypernatraemia
Hypocalcaemia
Hypomagnesaemia
Uraemia

Neurosurgical
Mass lesion in 'epileptogenic' area
Post-craniotomy haematoma
Head injury
Previous uncontrolled epilepsy

KEY POINTS

- Side-effects/interactions and plasma levels of anticonvulsant medication are important features.
- Careful choice of anaesthetic agents will allow intraoperative recording of spike activity.
- Risk of intraoperative and postoperative seizures.

FURTHER READING

Kofte WA, Templehoff R, Dasheiff RM. Anesthesia for epileptic patients and for epilepsy surgery. In: Cotteril JE, Smith DS (eds) Anesthesia for neurosurgery. St Louis: Mosby, 1994, p. 495

Modica PA, Tempelhoff R, White PF. Pro- and anticonvulsant effects of anaesthetics. (Part 1). Anesth Analg 1990; 70: 303

Modica PA, Tempelhoff R, White PF. Pro- and anticonvulsant effects of anaesthetics. (Part 2). Anesth Analg 1990; 70: 527

Smith M. Anaesthesia for epilepsy surgery. In: Shorvon SD, Dreifuss FE, Fish DF, Thomas DGT (eds) The treatment of epilepsy. Oxford: Blackwell Scientific, 1996

18

AWAKE CRANIOTOMY

M. Smith

INTRODUCTION

In the UK, most neurosurgical procedures are carried out under general anaesthesia. This allows for provision of optimal operating conditions with the ability to control $PaCO_2$ and blood pressure (BP) whilst assuring immobility and lack of awareness. Awake craniotomy is demanding for the neurosurgeon and neuroanaesthetist and requires a high degree of motivation from the patient.

BACKGROUND

The technique of awake craniotomy has developed over many years and initially involved local anaesthesia alone or combinations of local and general anaesthesia together with a variety of intraoperative wake-up techniques. The advent of neuroleptanaesthesia (e.g. using intravenous droperidol and opioids) offer some improvements in technique but the introduction of propofol presented an accurately titratable sedative with a rapid wake-up characteristic ideal for neurosurgical procedures.

PROCEDURES SUITABLE FOR AWAKE TECHNIQUES

- Epilepsy surgery.
- Stereotactic surgery.
- Functional surgery, e.g. pallidotomy, thalamotomy.
- Resection of mass lesions in eloquent areas (particularly in the dominant hemisphere).
- Cortical stimulation for recognition of motor, sensory and speech areas.
- Determination of memory and recognition areas (when combined with neuropsychological assessment).

PREOPERATIVE ASSESSMENT

Careful preoperative assessment and explanation are essential for success. It is crucial that the anaesthetist develops a good rapport with the patient and gives a detailed explanation of the procedure. In addition to routine preoperative considerations, the anaesthetist must decide whether the patient is sufficiently cooperative to participate in the procedure and whether they can tolerate lying supine and immobile for the duration of the operation.

INTRAOPERATIVE MANAGEMENT

All members of the theatre team must be briefed in advance so that a calm atmosphere prevails. It may be appropriate for patients to make their own selection of background music. Routine invasive cardiovascular monitoring is applied using local anaesthesia and a urinary catheter inserted if the procedure will be prolonged.

Some procedures, such as stereotactic brain biopsy, may be carried out entirely under local anaesthesia. More complex procedures, particularly those requiring craniotomy, are better suited to a combined technique of local anaesthesia and sedation.

Some form of airway management may be required during the sedation phase of the technique and in certain circumstances a laryngeal mask airway, which can be removed for the awake phase, may be suitable. There is a risk that the patient may cough during removal of the laryngeal mask and this is unacceptable in patients with an open dura. Furthermore, it can be difficult to re-insert the laryngeal mask should resedation be required during surgery.

An alternative option is to insert a soft nasopharyngeal airway into one nostril after preparation of the nasal mucosa with topical vasoconstrictor and local anaesthesia. This can safely remain in place throughout the procedure. It also has the advantage of allowing monitoring of end-tidal CO_2 by attachment of a side-stream CO_2 monitoring device into the end of the nasopharyngeal airway. Oxygen may be administered via the contralateral nostril.

The patient is transferred to the operating table and settled in a comfortable position prior to sedation. The head is best supported with a three-pin fixator applied using local anaesthesia (bupivacaine 0.5% with epinephrine). This prevents head movement during surgery and maximises airway control during the sedation phase. Surgical drapes are then positioned to allow continuous access by the anaesthetist to the patient and airway.

When the patient is comfortable, intravenous sedation is administered as appropriate. A small bolus of propofol followed by a titrated infusion works well, although more recently TCI propofol has been recommended. Patient-controlled sedation techniques with propofol may also be used. Incremental doses of a short-acting opioid such as fentanyl can be titrated against respiratory rate, but vigilance is required to prevent apnoea. Low dose remifentanil infusion is now a useful alternative. A small dose of droperidol (0.25–0.5 mg) minimises nausea during craniotomy.

When the patient is settled, local anaesthesia (0.5% bupivacaine with epinephrine) is applied to the skin and tissue layers down to the cranium, ensuring that the sensory nerves arising from the branches of the trigeminal nerve and cervical plexus are blocked. Although the skull has minimal sensation, raising the craniotomy flap can be an unpleasant experience because of noise from the power tools and incomplete anaesthesia. Sedation should therefore be continued until the dura is exposed. At this stage the dura is anaesthetised with plain lidocaine 1% by blocking the nerve trunk which runs with the middle meningeal artery and providing a field block around the edges of the craniotomy. The sedation should then be discontinued and the patient will rapidly regain consciousness and be able to participate in cortical stimulation testing. Furthermore, during epilepsy surgery, the EEG can be recorded awake without interference from anaesthetic agents (see Chapter 17).

Stimulation testing involves the application of a small electrical current to the cortex adjacent to the area of surgical interest. The resulting motor and sensory responses are used to map the cortical representation in that area, thereby allowing the neurosurgeon to determine the safe limits of the surgical resection. Despite cortical testing, many neurosurgeons prefer to complete the resection with the patient awake so that any infringement upon eloquent areas is immediately recognised. Following resection it is usually appropriate to re-sedate the patient during closure of the craniotomy.

INTRAOPERATIVE PROBLEMS

Although airway management is generally uneventful, sedation carries the risk of airway obstruction and apnoea. Facilities for emergency airway control should be available. The possibility of seizures also exists, particularly during cortical stimulation. Seizures should be terminated rapidly and a small bolus of propofol is usually adequate. The disadvantages of awake techniques include nausea, vomiting and difficulty in controlling blood pressure and $PaCO_2$. In patients undergoing epilepsy or functional surgery this is rarely a problem but, in patients with lesions causing a mass effect, brain swelling can be problematic.

POSTOPERATIVE CARE

This is determined by the neurosurgical procedure and there are no special requirements from the anaesthetic technique itself. Patients are fully alert and cooperative in the immediate postoperative period. Adequate analgesia should be provided before the effect of the local anaesthetic wears off.

KEY POINTS

- Patient cooperation is essential.
- Airway control during sedation phase is required.
- Sedation should continue until the dura is exposed.
- Seizures may occur, particularly with cortical stimulation.
- BP and $PaCO_2$ control may be difficult.
- Patients are fully alert and cooperative in the immediate postoperative period.

FURTHER READING

Herrick IA, Craen RA, Gelb AW, et al. Propofol sedation during awake craniotomy for seizures: electrocorticographic and epileptogenic effects. Anesth Analg 1997; 84: 1280

Huggins NJ. 'Diprifusor' for neurosurgical procedures. Anaesthesia 1998; 53 (suppl 1): 13

Johnson KB, Egan TD. Remifentanil and propofol combination for awake craniotomy: case report with pharmacokinetic simulations. J Neurosurg Anesthesiol 1998; 10: 25

Manninen P, Contreras J. Anesthetic considerations for craniotomy in awake patients. Int Anesthesiol Clin 1986; 24: 157

Smith M. Anaesthesia for epilepsy surgery. In: Shorvon SD, Dreifuss FE, Fish DF, Thomas DGT (eds). The treatment of epilepsy. Oxford: Blackwell Scientific, 1996

19

MICROVASCULAR DECOMPRESSION

K. Grixti

INTRODUCTION

Surgical decompression of cranial nerves near their root entry zones in the brainstem is considered when medical treatment has been unsuccessful, and may provide symptom relief from trigeminal neuralgia, hemifacial spasm and occasionally other conditions including glossopharyngeal neuralgia, tinnitus, positional vertigo, spastic torticollis, essential hypertension and intractable hiccups.

CLINICAL FEATURES

Trigeminal neuralgia is characterised by unilateral paroxysms of stabbing pain in one or more divisions of the trigeminal nerve territories. Often specific trigger zones or stimuli set off the pain many times a day. Occasionally multiple sclerosis or a benign tumour is the cause, however more commonly it is due to a small artery causing irritation of the root entry zone of CN V which can be seen by MR angiography.[2] It is more commonly seen in old age with atherosclerotic changes in the arteries. However, juvenile forms are sometimes seen with more severe anomalous vessel formation involving veins.

Hemifacial spasm is an irregular clonic spasm of the facial muscles usually involving one side of the face. Pain is not usually a feature unless fibres from the nervus intermedius are involved. The cause is usually secondary to aberrant blood vessels at the root entry zone of CN VII. It can be combined with other cranial nerve neuropathies commonly CN V and VIII. Other causes include acoustic neuroma, Paget's disease and following Bell's palsy.

Glossopharyngeal neuralgia is similar in aetiology and treatment. It manifests with paroxysms of pain at the back of the mouth and throat. Bradycardia and fainting may accompany the pain.

SURGICAL PROCEDURE

The surgery, known as the Janetta procedure, consists of inserting a muscle pad or Teflon sponge to separate the offending vessel and the nerve entry zone. It is performed via a retromastoid approach into the posterior fossa and usually takes 2–3 hours to complete. Recurrence of neuralgia after surgery may be due to slippage of the pad or due to reactive scar tissue which may also involve other cranial nerves.

The main surgical concern with microvascular decompression is damage to the auditory nerve secondary to stretching with the cerebellar retractor. Other possible mechanisms of damage include encroachment on the cochlear nucleus and vascular compromise leading to ischaemia. The incidence of complete hearing loss with trigeminal decompression is 1–4%, and up to 20% have partial hearing loss. Facial nerve decompression carries a higher risk due to the closer proximity of the nerve with the auditory nerve. Brainstem auditory evoked potentials intraoperatively reduces the incidence of postoperative deafness.

PREOPERATIVE MANAGEMENT

Medical treatment for trigeminal neuralgia consists of carbamazepine as a first-line drug or sodium valproate and phenytoin and all may interact with anaesthetic agents (see Chapter 11). These drugs must be continued and withdrawn gradually postoperatively to avoid rebound convulsions. Baclofen may also be used for trigeminal neuralgia and may cause bradycardia and hypotension with general anaesthetic agents.

INTRAOPERATIVE MANAGEMENT

Monitoring

Full monitoring should be used for all cases of posterior fossa surgery including direct arterial and venous pressure, end-tidal CO_2, pulse oximetry, electrocardiogram (ECG) and temperature.

Positioning

The patient is placed in the supine position, with the ipsilateral shoulder raised with a sandbag. The neck is flexed and rotated away from the operative side. Alternatively, the patient may be placed in the lateral or park bench position.

Anaesthesia

Anaesthesia is the same as for possa fossa surgery (see Chapter 14). Care must be taken with increased stimulation during laryngoscopy and intubation, pin placement from the skull pinholder, periosteal dissection, craniotomy and dural incision together with closure and headwrapping. Hypertensive responses can also be seen on manipulation of the trigeminal nerve while hypotension and bradycardia are seen with vagus nerve stimulation. Confirmation of airway and corneal reflexes immediately postoperatively is necessary.

ELECTROPHYSIOLOGICAL MONITORING

Somatosensory and trigeminal evoked potentials are sometimes used to monitor brainstem and trigeminal nerve function. In most cases the preoperative abnormality corrects itself during surgery, sometimes at the opening of the dura but mostly during dissection of the aberrant vessel. This gives a good indication of the likelihood of success of surgery.

Facial electromyography is used intraoperatively during CN VII decompression. This allows identification of aberrant vessels and correlates well with the success of surgery. The lateral spread response in facial EMG (i.e. the antidromic impulse in one facial nerve branch generated in response to a stimulus in another branch) resolves during decompression. Muscle relaxants are either not used or the twitch height kept at 30–40% of control. Caution must be exercised as surgical stimulation of motor centres at the brainstem may cause facial and shoulder movements.

Brainstem auditory evoked potenials involve recordings from scalp electrodes of the response to auditory clicks. An averaging technique involving over 2000 clicks eliminates background electrical activity of the scalp. This gives a typical 7 waveform response numbered from I to VII. Loss of amplitude of wave V is specific and has a high sensitivity in preventing surgical damage if measures to restore the wave are taken promptly. Concomitant direct compound action potentials on the exposed VIIIth nerve can help differentiate between damage to the acoustic nerve and cochlear nucleus.

KEY POINTS

- Microvascular decompression treats a range of cranial nerve neuropathies.
- These are mainly due to atherosclerotic vessels impinging on root entry zones in the brainstem.

- Separating the vessel and root entry zone by Teflon sponge is the most common surgical treatment.
- Complications include immediate cranial nerve neuropathies caused by surgical encroachment on the brainstem and delayed neuropathy caused by fibrosis around the sponge.
- Anaesthesia is the same as for posterior fossa surgery.
- Electrophysiological monitoring can be used to monitor surgical effectiveness and encroachment on neighbouring cranial nerves.

FURTHER READING

Gieger H, Naraghi R, Schobel HP, Frank H, Sterzel RB, Fahlbusch R. Decrease of blood pressure by ventromedullary decompression in essential hypertension. Lancet 1988; 352: 446

Mcaney JF, Eldridge PR, Dunn LT, Nixon TE, Whitehouse GT, Miles JB. Demonstration of neurovascular compression with MNR imaging. Comparison with surgical findings in 52 consecutive cases. J Neurosurg 1995; 83: 799

Resnick DK, Levy EI, Janetta PJ. Microvascular decompression for paediatric onset trigeminal neuralgia. Neurosurgery 1998; 32: 804

Hatayan T, Moeller AR. Correlation between latency and amplitude of peak V in the brain stem evoked potentials: intraoperative recording in microvascular decompression operation. Acta Neurosurg 1998; 140: 7

Moeller AR, Janetta PJ. Monitoring facial EMG responses during microvascular decompression operation for hemifacial spasm. J Neurosurg 1987; 66: 681

20

TRANSSPHENOIDAL HYPOPHYSECTOMY

R. Erskine, A. Summors

INTRODUCTION

Tumours of the pituitary region are common, accounting for 10–15% of intracranial neoplasms. An understanding of the anatomy, physiology and pathophysiology of the gland and its immediate relations is important in the management of patients for transsphenoidal surgery.

ANATOMY

The pituitary gland is situated in the upper aspect of the body of the sphenoid bone within the sella turcica. The bony floor of the sella consists of the roof of the sphenoid sinuses. The anterior tuberculum and the posterior dorsal wall are also sphenoid bone. Laterally on each side are the cavernous sinuses and their contents, the cranial nerves and the ICA (the arteries may indent the gland on each side). The roof of the sella (sella diaphragma) has dura mata attached to the anterior and posterior clinoid processes on each side. The hypophyseal stalk acting as a conduit for nerves and the vessels of the portal system descending from the hypothalamus, pierces this dura. A wide dural opening may lead to transmission of CSF pressure giving rise eventually to the empty sella syndrome. The optic nerves converge above the sella to form the optic chiasm.

PHYSIOLOGY

The gland has two distinct components. The anterior pituitary (*adenohypophysis*) releases hormones (Table 20.1) in pulsatile fashion that regulate growth and development, thyroid function, the adrenal cortex, breast and gonads. The secretion of these hormones are directed by releasing hormones formed in the hypothalamus and conveyed to the gland by the pituitary portal vessels.

The posterior pituitary (*neurohypophysis*) is responsible for the release of vasopressin, oxytocin and antidiuretic hormone. These octapeptides are carried down to the pituitary from the hypothalamus in secretory granules along nervous tissue within the pituitary stalk by an active transport mechanism.

PATHOPHYSIOLOGY

Functioning tumours derived from the adenohypophysis may secrete excess hormone to impinge on anaesthetic management of the patient undergoing surgical resection. Excesses of adrenocorticotropic hormone (ACTH) and growth hormone (GH) only, present management problems (see below). Prolactin hypersecretion is present in 60% of all cases due to the failure of the normal hypothalamic suppression of prolactin secretion. Prolactinomas are usually first

---

Table 20.1 Hypothalamic release and inhibiting hormones controlling anterior pituitary hormone release

Anterior pituitary hormone	Release hormone	Inhibiting hormone
ACTH	Corticoliberin* (corticotrophin releasing factor)	
GH	Somatoliberin* (GH releasing factor)	Somatostatin* (GH release inhibiting hormone)
PRL	Thyroliberin* (thyrotropin releasing hormone)	Prolactostatin* (prolactin release inhibiting hormone)
TSH	Thyroliberin*	Somatostatin*
LH	Folliberin* (gonadotrophin releasing hormone)	
FSH	Folliberin*	
MSH	Melanoliberin* (melanotropin releasing hormone)	Melanostatin* (melanotropin release inhibiting hormone)

* Recommended by IUPAC-IUB Committee on Biochemical Nomenclature 1974

treated medically with bromocriptine. Up to 30% of pituitary adenomas are endocrinologically silent and present with symptoms secondary to mass effects (headache, visual field disturbance) or pituitary hypofunction secondary to destruction of normal gland. Parasellar tumours may also present this way. The most common are craniopharyngiomas formed from the embryonic remains of Rathke's pouch (the origin of the anterior pituitary). Other tumours in this area include meningiomas and gliomas of the optic chiasma.

Increasing tumour pressure produces failure of hormone secretion in a typical order, i.e. gonadotrophins first, followed by GH, ACTH and thyroid-stimulating hormone (TSH). A patient presenting for surgery with normal gonadal function will consequently not be deficient in any other pituitary hormone.

GH AND ACROMEGALY

Acromegaly commonly gives rise to diabetes mellitus and all patients exhibit an abnormal glucose tolerance. Hypertension and coronary artery disease is usually present. Patients may present with a cardiomyopathy leading to cardiomegaly and failure. The most notable changes are in the bones and soft tissues of the face with enlargement and thickening within these structures. Airway difficulties are produced by an enlarged tongue and soft tissue hypertrophy within the pharynx. Narcolepsy and sleep apnoea are common. The degree of airway compromise may require an awake fibreoptic intubation to avoid the need for tracheostomy.

ACTH AND CUSHING'S DISEASE

Most of these tumours are ACTH-secreting microadenomas (less than 10 mm diameter). Features of the disease result from secondary adrenal hyperplasia. These features are both physical and physiological. Physical features include truncal obesity, osteoporosis and kyphosis (the so-called buffalo hump). Hypertension and glucose intolerance nearly always features, although frank diabetes is unusual. Depression is also common. Patients may receive metyrapone, a metabolic inhibitor of cortisol synthesis prior to surgery. These patients need cortisol supplementation perioperatively. Postoperatively a synacthen test is performed to test for residual deficiency of cortisol response.

PITUITARY APOPLEXY

Tumours of the pituitary may suddenly enlarge as a result of bleeding with consequent infarction and necrosis of the tumour and possibly the whole pituitary. The signs are those of meningism with or without sudden blindness. SAH may be a feature. This constitutes a surgical emergency and surgery must take place within hours. Patients should be supplemented with steroids intraoperatively. Panhypopituitarism may be a feature.

DIABETES INSIPIDUS

Diabetes insipidus (DI) may be a feature of patients presenting for transsphenoidal surgery. Polyuria results from insufficient synthesis or release of antidiuretic hormone (ADH). In addition, surgery in this region often (in about 50% of cases) results in a temporary state of DI postoperatively. Glucocorticoids and mineralocorticoids are necessary for the control of fluid balance. DI may not manifest in anterior pituitary insufficiency until the patient is supplemented with steroids. Section of the pituitary stalk produces temporary DI that resolves with time as ADH is released into the blood directly from the median eminence. In the postoperative period, close attention should be paid to fluid balance and osmolality. Supplementation with the synthetic ADH analogue Desmopressin (DDAVP) should be cautious anticipating a return of endogenous ADH.

PREOPERATIVE MANAGEMENT

Anaesthetic management of patients for transsphenoidal surgery is similar to transcranial surgery. The patient should undergo appropriate preoperative investigation and preparation, including baseline endocrine function tests and investigation of anatomical manifestations (e.g. changes in airway). The preoperative visit ascertains the general patient condition with particular attention to anatomical or metabolic consequences of pituitary pathology. An enlarged tongue in acromegaly may make intubation more difficult. Any medical treatment is continued into the postoperative period. Assessment of the hypothalmic–pituitary axis will establish the requirement for glucocorticoid replacement. Thyroid function should be controlled and diabetes stabilised. Antibiotic prophylaxis is commonly given especially for at risk patients (those with nasal or sinus infections, previous pituitary surgery and Cushing's syndrome).

Explanations are given for mouthbreathing postoperatively, intensive care admission, or awake fibreoptic intubation if required.

A short-acting benzodiazepine is sufficient for premedication if required.

INTRAOPERATIVE MANAGEMENT

The patient is positioned either supine with the head extended or semi-recumbent with the head slightly to the right. The guiding C arm of the image intensifier is positioned for a lateral view to guide the surgeon. The anaesthetist and their equipment are positioned along one side of the patient.

Anaesthetic aims are a smooth induction, stable maintenance and recovery with appropriate monitoring and fluid management with control of ICP but it is rare to have raised ICP without suprasellar extension. Anaesthesia is routinely induced using an intravenous induction agent, opioid analgesic and non-depolarising muscle relaxant of choice. Invasive arterial monitoring is recommended. An oral armoured endotracheal tube is taped securely out of the left-hand side of the mouth and a throat pack inserted.

Good venous access is important. Bleeding is usually minimal but when it occurs, it may be catastrophic. Central venous access is not usually required unless indicated for the patient's medical condition.

Maintenance of anaesthesia can be achieved with a total intravenous technique or with inhalational agents with or without N_2O. Dissection and drilling to the sella can be highly stimulating and an infusion of remifentanil at this stage has proven helpful. Valsava manoeuvres on occasion may be required to prolapse the gland down, or check for leaks of CSF at the end of surgery. A mean BP between 60 and 80 mmHg at the highest point of the skull maintains CPP and minimises blood in the surgical field.

At the end of surgery the nose is comprehensively packed to prevent bleeding and the patient is woken ensuring the throat pack is removed. Fluid balance is observed closely in the postoperative period. Opioid analgesia may be required postoperatively although care must be taken to avoid respiratory depression.

KEY POINTS

- An understanding of the anatomy and pathophysiology of pituitary tumours is essential for their management.
- Tumours may produce hormones or be nonfunctioning and produce mass effects or destroy normal pituitary tissue.
- Excess GH or ACTH requires careful anaesthetic management.
- DI may be a significant problem in the perioperative period.

FURTHER READING

Matjasko MJ. Anesthetic considerations in patients with endocrine disease. In: Cottrell JE, Smith DS (eds) Anesthesia and neurosurgery. St Louis: Mosby, 1994, pp. 604–624

Jewkes D. Anaesthesia for pituitary surgery. Curr Anaes Crit Care 1993; 4: 8–12

Drury PL. Endocrinology. In: Kumar P, Clark (eds) Clinical medicine, 3rd Edn. London: Bailliére-Tindall, 1994, pp. 769–824

Landolt AM, Schiller Z. Surgical technique: transsphenoidal approach. In: Landolt AM, Vance ML, Reilly PL (eds) Pituitary adenomas. London: Churchill-Livingstone, 1966, p. 315

21

STEREOTACTIC SURGERY

A. Summors

INTRODUCTION

Image-guided stereotactic surgery allows access to intracranial lesions without the need for craniotomy enabling safer biopsy of very small lesions and lesions close to vital centres. Stereotaxis can also be used to choose the craniotomy site for minimal access surgery such as the removal of secondary tumour deposits on the surface of the brain or for the delivery of radiotherapy via CT-guided radioactive wires.

A mechanical frame is attached to the patient's head and a CT scan obtained. The scanner's computer calculates the 3-D coordinates of points in the brain and relates them to the stereotactic space outlined by the frame. Simple calculations convert these radiographic coordinates to the coordinate system used by the frame. These coordinates are set on the micrometers on the frame through which biopsy instruments can be directed with an accuracy of 1–2 mm.

Alternatively, *frameless stereotaxy* allows surgeons to reassess direction and approach to surgery without having to repeat imaging of the brain to establish new 3-D coordinates. The initial CT or MR image is stored on computer in the operating theatre and fixed points on the skull are mapped onto the image using a sensor wand. The tip of the sensor can then define the lesion on all axes of interest on CT, MRI or fused images of both.

ANAESTHESIA

External frame systems require the use of metal pins to fix the frame to the head. These can be applied under local anaesthesia supplemented with sedation if required. The burrhole for biopsy can also be performed under local anaesthesia. This has the advantage of continuous patient evaluation during transfer between the radiology suite and operating theatre and during biopsy.

General anaesthesia, however, is more common especially for prolonged procedures and for children. The patient is anaesthetised prior to application of the frame and CT scan and then transferred anaesthetised to the operating theatre for burrhole biopsy.

Patients who are otherwise fit and do not require invasive monitoring may be induced within the radiology suite. The essential criteria to perform general anaesthesia outside the operating theatre are outlined in Table 21.1.

Patients with multi-system disease requiring invasive monitoring for safe anaesthesia should be induced in the operating theatre, transferred to the radiology suite and returned back to theatre.

Table 21.1 Criteria for general anaesthesia outside the operating theatre
1. Reliable source of oxygen.
2. Portable means of manually and mechanically ventilating patient
3. Intubating equipment to place an armoured endotracheal tube. (A laryngeal mask airway is useful for unexpected difficult intubation in the X-ray department.)
4. Portable monitoring including ECG, NIBP and pulse oximetry. Capnography is desirable but not essential.
5. Immediate access to all drugs that may be required.
6. Patient on bed or trolley capable of immediate head down tilt.
7. Working portable suction apparatus.

The anaesthetic technique is aimed at cardiovascular and respiratory stability to maintain a stable CPP and ICP, minimising oedema and consequent lesion movement with respect to the skull.

A total intravenous system utilising propofol to induce and maintain anaesthesia is commonly used. This avoids the need for an anaesthetic machine during transfer and problems of pollution with scavenging of inhalational agents. Propofol can be used to ease the stimulus of siting the stereotactic frame and allows fast recovery if the procedure to follow requires the patient to be awake, e.g. thalamotomy. A modest dose of short-acting narcotic may also be used together with monitored muscle relaxation. The same anaesthetic technique can be continued in the operating room.

All monitors, pumps, O_2 cylinders and ventilator should be fixed securely to the transfer trolley and arranged for easy observation from outside the CT scanner. Good venous access should be secured as the biopsy may provoke bleeding which may be fatal.

KEY POINTS

- Stereotactic surgery usually requires anaesthesia in a site remote from the operating room.
- A total intravenous technique based on propofol, opioid and muscle relaxation provides stability, adequate depth of anaesthesia for all stages of stereotaxis and a rapid reliable recovery.

FURTHER READING

Salcman M. The surgical management of gliomas. In: Tindall GT, Cooper PR, Barrow PL (eds) The practice of neurosurgery. Baltimore: Williams & Wilkins, 1996, pp. 649–670

Bone ME, Bristow A. Total intravenous anaesthesia in stereotactic surgery: one years clinical experience. Eur J Anaesthesiol 1991; 8: 47–54

Powell M. Recent advances: neurosurgery. Br Med J 1999; 318: 35–38

22

ANAESTHESIA FOR HEAD INJURY

C. Duffy

INTRODUCTION

Over one million people present to hospital each year in the UK with head injury (HI) and, of these, over half are aged under 16 years. HI occurs twice as often in males and peaks from teenage years up to 40 years old. In the UK, 15–20% of all deaths in the 15 to 35-year age group are due to head injury.

The main causes of HI are falls (41%), assaults (20%) and road traffic accidents (RTAs) (13%). RTAs are associated with more severe injuries and account for 58% of all deaths from HI.

The GCS is used as a guide to severity of HI after hypovolaemia, hypoxia, drug and alcohol effects have been corrected. On the basis of GCS, HI severity can be divided into mild (GCS 13–15), moderate (GCS 9–12) or severe (GCS < 8) injury.

Although little can be done to repair the neural damage from the *primary injury*, the *secondary injury* which occurs as a result of additional mechanical or metabolic derangement triggered by the primary event may be amenable to medical intervention. Secondary injury may be systemic or intracranial in origin (Table 22.1). Systemic and CNS monitoring allow for early detection and prompt treatment of factors that may exacerbate secondary injury.

Associated injuries occur in half of severe HIs and evidence for these should be sought particularly involving spine (2–5% of severe HIs), chest (e.g. cardiac tamponade, contusion, pneumothorax), abdomen, pelvis and limb fractures. In cases of multi-trauma, injuries need to be prioritised appropriately.

INDICATIONS FOR SURGICAL MANAGEMENT

The following sequelae need urgent neurosurgical intervention:

Table 22.1 Systemic and intracranial causes of secondary brain injury

Systemic causes	Intracranial causes
Hypotension, acidosis, hypoxia, hypoglycaemia, hyperglycaemia, hyperthermia, coagulopathy, sepsis, anaemia.	Intracranial hypertension, oedema, vasospasm, infection, epilepsy

1. *Skull fractures* depressed greater than skull thickness. Compound fractures with torn dura need repair to reduce infection risk.
2. *Intracranial mass lesions* with > 5 mm midline shift or basal cistern compression on CT scan (i.e. a sign of imminent transtentorial herniation).
3. Most *acute subdural* and *epidural haematomas* need evacuation within 2–4 hours of injury to achieve optimal chance of recovery.
4. *Intracerebral haematoma*: The decision to operate is guided by the patient's clinical condition and ICP. Urgent surgical management is required for large temporal lobe lesions (due to risk of transtentorial herniation) and posterior fossa collections (causing brainstem compression).
5. *Refractory intracranial hypertension* may improve with decompressive craniectomy.
6. *Delayed hydrocephalus* occurs in 6% of severe HIs, usually 14 days post-injury.

PATHOPHYSIOLOGY

1. *Haemorrhagic contusions* are superficial multiple bilateral areas of haemorrhage usually affecting grey matter of temporal and frontal lobes. They account for 3% of severe head injuries. The CT image is characterised by a 'salt and pepper' appearance due to interspersed haemorrhage and oedema. Contusions are better delineated with MRI scans.
2. *Intracerebral haematomas* usually affect the white matter or basal ganglia and are the cause of delayed neurological deterioration in 8–19% of patients admitted with severe HI. Haematoma is differentiated from contusion by demarcation between normal and injured brain. The prognosis is usually good unless there is a marked mass effect.
3. *Subdural haematomas (SDH)* are due to tearing of cortical veins between the dura and pia arachnoid and appear crescent-shaped on CT scan occurring most commonly in the inferior frontal and anterior temporal lobes. They can be classified as acute (< 3–4 days old and appearing hyperdense on CT imaging), subacute (4–20 days old, isodense) and chronic (> 20 days old, hypodense) and are predisposed with increasing age, alcoholism, coagulopathy, epilepsy and in those with ventricular shunts. A poor outcome is more likely if SDH is bilateral, accumulates rapidly, or there is a > 4 hour delay in surgical management of acute SDH. Increased patient age and underlying brain contusion also lead to poor outcome.
4. *Extradural haematomas (EDH)* are biconvex lenticular lesions between the skull and dura. Most

(90%) are associated with skull fractures and due to injury of the middle meningeal artery and therefore affect the parietal and parieto-temporal areas. The remainder is due to venous sinus laceration. Underlying brain contusion is less common than with SDH. Outcome depends on the level of consciousness at the time of surgery with mortality approaching 20% if unconscious.

5. *Diffuse axonal injury (DAI)* occurs in 50–60% of severe head injuries and is characterised by small bilateral non-haemorrhagic lesions affecting the lobar white matter, corpus callosum and upper brainstem. They are classified as mild (coma for 6–24 hours), moderate (> 24 hours coma without decerebrate posturing) and severe (> 24 hours coma with decerebrate posturing). Outcome is usually poor with the mortality for severe DAI approaching 50%.

6. *Traumatic arterial and venous injuries* (e.g. dissection, fistula formation, pseudoaneurysm) are diagnosed by angiography. These injuries may be associated with subarachnoid haemorrhage and secondary vasospasm.

PREOPERATIVE MANAGEMENT

History

An accurate account of the acute injury is important in assessment. Progressive loss of consciousness suggests an expanding intracranial mass. If the patient has been unconscious from the time of accident, DAI is likely.

Resuscitation

The initial resuscitation and transfer is described in Chapter 37.

INTRAOPERATIVE MANAGEMENT

Monitoring should include ECG, pulse oximetry, capnography, invasive pressure monitoring, arterial blood gases, $SjvO_2$, glucose, electrolytes, haematocrit and coagulation. The aims of intraoperative management are similar to those for elective craniotomy (Chapter 12), with some notable additions:

- Brain swelling is likely and a target CPP > 70 mmHg should be maintained. Commencement of inotropes may be required.
- Hyperventilation below $PaCO_2$ of 4 kPa should be avoided and $SjvO_2$ should remain above 50%. Patients should be paralysed and have adequate analgesia. The choice of anaesthetic agent is not a crucial factor, although inhalational agents should

be used in concentrations < 1 MAC, and nitrous oxide is best avoided. $CMRO_2$ should be minimised and an infusion of propofol is often useful. The use of mild hypothermia (33–35°C) is controversial but frequently used.

Normovolaemia, an appropriate haematocrit for the patient's age and underlying medical condition and a normal blood sugar should be maintained. Hypotonic and glucose-containing solutions should be avoided and there is some evidence in favour of using *hypertonic* solutions.

COMPLICATIONS

Up to 20% of patients with acute SDH develop sudden and massive brain swelling at the time of clot removal. This should be treated with increased ventilation (ensuring $SjvO_2 > 50\%$), diuretics (mannitol or furosemide) and removal of CSF. Administration of thiopentone or propofol to achieve EEG burst suppression should be considered. Swollen brain tissue may need to be retracted (leading to further injury) or resected.

Penetrating brain injuries may be associated with profuse bleeding, usually from venous sinuses. Post-traumatic seizures occur in 15% of severe head injuries and are treated with phenytoin for up to 1 week post-injury.

POSTOPERATIVE MANAGEMENT

Continued sedation and ventilation with ICP monitoring is required for low preoperative GCS and for multiple associated injuries. Extubated patients need to be monitored closely in a dependent setting for neurological deterioration. Postoperative rises in ICP may be due to local swelling or development of a new lesion and occurs more commonly following evacuation of intracerebral haematoma.

KEY POINTS

- Hypotension must be avoided by adequate fluid resuscitation.
- Consider associated injuries. Chest injuries may cause hypoxia which must be avoided.
- A stable anaesthetic is required, with manipulation of intracranial physiology in order to maintain CPP > 70 mmHg.
- Neuroprotective strategies such as EEG burst suppression with intravenous anaesthetic agents, may be required.

- Postoperative high dependency or intensive care with ICP monitoring is essential.

FURTHER READING

Polin RS, Shaffrey ME, Bogaev CA, et al. Decompressive bifrontal craniectomy in the treatment of severe refractory posttraumatic cerebral edema. Neurosurgery 1997; 41: 84–94

Gopinath SP, Robertson CS. Management of severe head injury. In: Cottrell JE, Smith DS (eds) Anesthesia and neurosurgery. St Louis: Mosby, 1994, pp. 661–684

The Royal College of Surgeons of England. Report of the working party on the management of patients with head injuries. London: RCSE, 1999

McGrath BJ, Matjasko J. Anaesthesia and head trauma. New Horizons 1995; 3: 523–533

23

COMPLEX CERVICAL SPINE SURGERY

I. Calder

INTRODUCTION

Cervical spinal cord disease due to extrinsic causes such as compression results from both a combination of cord *deformation* and the *duration* of deformation. Improvements in axonal survival by limiting cord deformation and duration of deformation may have clinical benefit (e.g. after experimental trauma in animals, those with preserved function had greater numbers of surviving neurones). The damage to the cord results from hypoperfusion, which suggests that patients with severe cervical disease undergoing long, complicated surgery are likely to be at greater risk. The contribution of hypoperfusion to spinal cord injury (SCI) during anaesthesia has been under-estimated, although there has been an over-emphasis on mechanical trauma due to direct laryngoscopy.

PRACTICAL CONSIDERATIONS

An increased risk of neurological deterioration during surgery on the cervical spine exists with:

1. Poor pre-operative neurological function
2. Instrumentation
3. Upper cervical and clival surgery
4. Multisegmental surgery
5. Prolonged hypotension

DIRECT LARYNGOSCOPY

Clear evidence that direct laryngoscopy has produced SCI is lacking. The procedure is generally of short duration, involves little spinal movement below C2 and raises spinal cord perfusion pressure (SCPP). Most reports alleging that SCI was due to direct laryngoscopy have come from non-anaesthetic authors.

POSITIONING

Abnormal positioning (excessive flexion or extension) for prolonged periods (typically > 8 hours) may cause SCI in patients with normal cervical spine. However, there have been reports of SCI with shorter periods of surgery. Positioning patients for protracted surgery is largely guesswork; evoked potential monitoring is currently the best guide to whether a position is being tolerated (see below).

PERFUSION PRESSURE

Blood flow through healthy arteries of the brain and spinal cord is autoregulated to remain constant over a range of blood pressures. Very low MAP has resulted in ischaemic damage to the cord in patients with *normal* spines. In spinal cord disease, auto-regulation is unreliable so that even moderate falls in pressure may reduce perfusion. Maintenance of MAP at levels that should ensure an adequate SCPP (about 70 mmHg) is a sensible precaution. This should be continued in the postoperative period and may require the use of inotropes. Perfusion may also be compromised if the CSF pressure is high. CSF pressure can vary with position and alignment of the spine. The measurement and adjustment by drainage of CSF pressure through a lumbar intrathecal catheter is logical during major cervical surgery but in practice, case selection is problematic, since insertion of the catheter is difficult in such patients and the procedure has considerable morbidity. The use of induced hypertension to ensure an adequate SCPP may be beneficial, but carries the risk of increased oedema and haemorrhage in the damaged spinal cord. Pharmacological spinal cord protection with NMDA receptor blockers (e.g. Mg^{++}) has shown promise in animal studies.

SPINAL CORD MONITORING DURING ANAESTHESIA

General anaesthesia abolishes the clinical signs of myelopathy - weakness, sensory and reflex changes.

1. *Observation of pulse and blood pressure:* SCI produced by experimental trauma to the cervical cord of animals produces initial hypertension, followed by hypotension and bradycardia. Although these haemodynamic changes are seen in humans, they are not a constant feature and severe damage may occur without these signs being apparent.
2. *Avoidance of neuro-muscular blockade during anaesthesia:* Surgical stimulation of the cord or nerve root may produce movement in a limb, which is a useful warning. Immobility during general anaesthesia is largely due to abolition of spinal reflexes; brainstem destruction has little effect on MAC. An opioid infusion (e.g. fentanyl or remifentanil) and ventilation with approximately one MAC of a volatile agent provides satisfactory conditions.
3. *Sensory evoked potential monitoring:* Sensory evoked potentials can be monitored by detecting the cortical response to a peripheral stimulus (see Chapter 57). The median nerve is used for monitoring cervical cord function. Sensory potentials demonstrate continuity of the sensory not the motor tracts, but serious damage to the motor tracts without alteration of sensory responses is unusual.

4. *Motor evoked potential monitoring:* Demonstration of intact motor pathways throughout anaesthesia is attractive, but more difficult in practice than sensory monitoring.
5. *Local anaesthesia:* More spinal surgery could be performed under local anaesthesia than at present, but special characteristics are probably required of patient and surgeon.

AIRWAY MANAGEMENT

The method of airway management is influenced by the patient's neurological condition, the site of surgery, and the likelihood of the need for re-intubation

Tracheostomy

This is often the most sensible option in patients with anteriorly placed lesions at the cranio-cervical junction. Tracheostomy should be considered in patients with severe high cervical myelopathy.

Tracheal intubation

Difficult tracheal intubation can be expected with cranio-cervical junction disease, fixation devices, flexion deformity and temporo-mandibular joint disease. Flexible fibreoptic technology provides the best conditions in difficult cases and the nasal route is usually easiest, due to the favourable 'angle of attack' and lack of gagging in awake patients (see Chapter 24). Nasal tubes should not remain for more than a few days, because of the risk of sinusitis.

Extubation

The timing of extubation in patients who are known to be difficult to intubate, and particularly those who may be difficult to mask-ventilate is important. These patients should be extubated during normal working hours, be normothermic, cardiovascularly stable, with satisfactory gas exchange and acid/base balance, and be neurologically stable.

Anterior cervical haematoma

Typically, a surgical collar hides the haematoma post operatively. The patient complains of not being able to breathe, and stridor and desaturation are late signs. The wound should be opened immediately and blood clot expressed. Induction of anaesthesia is dangerous as swelling of the soft tissues around the glottis may make mask-ventilation and intubation impossible. An inhalational induction is recommended.

POSITIONING FOR SURGERY

The head is commonly held by a skull pin device such as the Mayfield™ frame. Insertion of these pins is extremely painful and profound analgesia is required, which can result in a period of hypotension if pin insertion is delayed. Inotropic support may be necessary.

The eyes are at risk, particularly with the prone position. The eye must be closed and waterproofed to prevent damage due to skin preparation fluids and blood. Rarer causes of eye damage include ischaemic optic neuropathy and retinal vessel thrombosis.

Posterior approaches

A posterior approach requires the prone or sitting position, both of which are problematic for the anaesthetist. From a surgical perspective, the posterior approach is relatively uncomplicated, since the airway and major blood vessels are not in the way. However, lesions anterior to the cord are not easily accessible from the back of the neck and retraction of the spinal cord is dangerous.

Anterior approaches

Anterior lesions around the cranio-cervical junction may necessitate extensive surgery, since access is impeded by the maxilla superiorly and the mandible and tongue inferiorly. Localised lesions can be reached by a trans-oral approach, but lesions extending up or down may require a maxillotomy or mandibular and tongue split. These operations involve problems with the management of the airway and nutrition. Anterior lesions below C2/3 are relatively easily accessed, but there is a risk of damage to the trachea, pharynx, oesophagus, carotid vessels and the vagus or recurrent laryngeal nerves. Postoperative haematoma may cause airway obstruction.

Lateral approaches

There is a risk of bleeding from the vertebral artery.

NUTRITION

Swallowing is frequently difficult after anterior cervical surgery.

Surgery below C2

It can prove extremely difficult to insert a naso-gastric tube in the intubated patient in whom laryngoscopy has been difficult. The tube should be inserted *before* the patient is anaesthetised if a difficult laryngoscopy is expected. A nasogastric tube should also be inserted if extensive surgery is contemplated. This can be removed when the patient can swallow. A tube should also be placed if the pharynx or oesophagus is perforated during surgery.

Trans-oral maxillotomy, Mandibulotomy with tongue split

Serious consideration should be given to the insertion of a percutaneous gastrostomy (PEG) before such surgery. A PEG should always be inserted when the tongue is split, since swallowing takes some weeks to recover. Nasogastric tubes have proved to be better tolerated than feeding pharyngostomies in our experience, but the risk of infection makes prolonged nasogastric intubation unwelcome when there is a pharyngeal wound, particularly when the dura has been breached.

Postoperative care

Surgery requiring fusion or instrumentation frequently requires a hard collar to prevent excessive movement initially. Opiate analgesia is usually necessary particularly if a bone graft has been taken. Antiemetic administration is essential to avoid the risk of vomiting on emergence.

KEY POINTS

- Spinal cord damage is due to a combination of degree and duration of cord compression.
- Attention to positioning is essential to prevent cord injury, particularly during prolonged surgery.
- Careful consideration regarding airway management is required preoperatively.
- Maintenance of cord perfusion pressure is essential.
- Coughing and vomiting at the end of surgery should be avoided.

FURTHER READING

Calder l, Calder J, Crockard HA. Difficult direct laryngoscopy in patients with cervical spine disease. Anaesthesia 1995; 50: 756-63

McLeod ADM, Calder I. Spinal cord injury and direct laryngoscopy – the legend lives on. Br J Anaes 2000; 84: 705–9.

Singh U, Silver JR, Welply NC. Hypotensive infarction of the spinal cord. Paraplegia 1994; 32: 314-22

Vale FL, Burns J, Jackson AB, Hadley MN. Combined medical and surgical treatment after acute spinal cord injury: results of a prospective pilot study to assess the merits of aggressive medical resuscitation and blood pressure management. J Neurosurg 1997; 87: 239-46

Slucky AV. Acute spinal cord injuries. The Cervical Spine Research Society Editorial Committee. The Cervical Spine. 3rd ed [52], 521-39. Philadelphia: Lippincott-Raven Publishers. 1998

24

FIBREOPTIC INTUBATION

I. Calder

INTRODUCTION

Flexible fibreoptic technology allows inspection and intubation of the trachea under vision, and since the introduction of an endoscope is well tolerated by patients, a tracheal airway can be placed before the induction of general anaesthesia. Easy endoscopy requires:

1. An air space
2. Minimal secretions
3. Good patient preparation
4. Experience and familiarity with the anatomy of the airway
5. Time.

Endoscopy may be of limited use in some difficult airway situations, particularly during emergencies where there is swelling, displacement and deformation of tissue, bleeding and secretions. It is most successful as an elective procedure in conditions in which airway access is diminished by poor craniocervical extension or mouth opening.

IDENTIFICATION OF PATIENTS REQUIRING FLEXIBLE FIBREOPTIC INTUBATION

It is easy to identify patients that obviously require fibreoptic intubation. Identifying the less obvious patient remains more of an art than a science.

RHEUMATOID ARTHRITIS

Patients suffering from cervical rheumatoid disease are frequently difficult to laryngoscope directly. Glottic involvement is common (patients will often admit to intermittent hoarseness and stridor). Fibreoptic intubation has been shown to reduce the incidence of post-extubation stridor in these patients.

UNSTABLE CERVICAL SPINE

The advantage of fibreoptic intubation over direct laryngoscopy with regards to neurological safety is unproven. No convincing report of cervical spinal cord injury due to direct laryngoscopy has appeared. However, the lack of published evidence of direct laryngoscopy-induced cord injury can not be taken as proof that the procedure is without hazard; difficult direct laryngoscopy is hazardous for normal patients, and cervical disease should militate against any attempt at direct laryngoscopy that involves more than minimal force.

Many 'unstable' cervical spines have been rendered rigid by the application of fixation devices, such as halo-body frames, when presented for anaesthesia. In these circumstances, flexible fibreoptic intubation is the best option.

CONDUCT OF FIBREOPTIC INTUBATION

Successful fibreoptic intubation depends on:

- Orientation
- Vision
- Ventilation
- Suppression (of reflexes)
- Sedation
- Position
- Rotation (of the tracheal tube).

ORIENTATION

The commonest cause of difficulty is that the endoscopist loses their orientation. If a television system is used it is essential to establish that the screen view corresponds to the eyepiece view. It will be helpful to know where the top, bottom and sides of the airway are to be found as the endoscope is advanced, as identification of anatomy (particularly abnormal anatomy) is then much more likely. Loss of orientation is nearly always the result of failing to identify the hard palate (nasal approach) or tongue (oral approach). With the nasal approach, it is useful to identify the hard palate *before entering the nostril*. It is sensible to examine both nostrils and choose the more patent. Once the palate is identified, it is simple to follow it, turn over or under the soft palate (depending on the position of the endoscopist), enter the oro-pharynx and identify glottic structures. With an oral approach, the fibreoptic laryngoscope is kept in the midline with the tongue at the top or bottom of the field.

VISION

Adequate vision depends on an air space and minimal secretions. Provision of an air space and minimisation of secretions are the objectives. An awake patient has the most patent airway. Artificial airways such as the Ovassapian or COPA can be helpful, whilst the LMA nearly always provides a satisfactory view.

The administration of drying agents is not usually necessary, but is essential if topical anaesthesia is to be effective. Secretions can be 'blown away' by insufflation of oxygen through the suction channel, but rupture of the stomach has been reported. In the awake patient asking for a deep breath is usually very helpful. The LMA (or ILMA) is particularly useful when there are copious secretions, since they help to isolate the glottis from secretions. The suction channel in fibreoptic laryngoscopes is ineffective; a normal suction catheter is better.

VENTILATION

Anxiety about ventilation of the anaesthetised patient will distract the endoscopist. Relative inexperience in endoscopy (of both operator and assistants) should be regarded as reasons to consider an awake endoscopy. There are two options:

1. *Apnoea:* The experienced endoscopist will be able to intubate an apnoeic patient in much the same time as is required with direct laryngoscopy.
2. *Ventilation systems:* Artificial aids to ventilation in anaesthetised patients include special face masks, nasal airways, modified Guedel airways and the COPA. The LMA and ILMA provide the most satisfactory solution to the problem of ventilation during endoscopy. Ventilation of the patient's lungs can continue whilst the endoscope is inserted through a bronchoscopic catheter mount. The endoscope is withdrawn when the operator is confident of entry to the trachea, the catheter mount is removed and the endoscope re-inserted.

A crico-thyroid cannula can provide a means of ventilation, and be placed before induction of anaesthesia. It is essential that intra-tracheal placement is confirmed before insufflation with high airway pressures.

SUPPRESSION OF REFLEXES

Coughing, breath holding and laryngospasm are all frequent problems during endoscopy in anaesthetised patients with normal neuromuscular transmission. Neuromuscular blockade solves these problems, but ability to ventilate the lungs should be ensured before the agent is given.

Suppression of the glottic reflexes with local anaesthetic agents is easily performed in elective cases. Lidocaine works better (and is absorbed better) if the mucosa is dry. A drying agent such as glycopyrrolate should be given, preferably at least 30 minutes before the start. Lidocaine is relatively free from toxic complications when applied to the nasopharynx and glottis but is distinctly irritant. Minor degrees of stridor are not uncommon and complete airway obstruction has been reported. Doses up to 10 mg/kg of lidocaine are acceptable, but hypotension is sometimes seen following intubation. The use of the oral route in awake patients is complicated by the gag reflex, which follows stimulation of the base of the tongue. Blockade of the lingual branch of the glossopharyngeal nerve may partially obtund this reflex, but needle insertion is difficult if the patient cannot open their mouth adequately, as is usual. Topical 10% lidocaine spray directed to the distal paraglossal gutter may be more reliable than a needle blockade of the nerve. The use of a dental prop is recommended if the oral route is used in an awake patient.

The nasal route avoids the gag reflex and provides a better angle of attack. In preparation, 2% lidocaine gel should be instilled into the nasal cavity, followed by 10% spray into the oropharynx. Vasoconstrictors such as xylometazoline and phenylephrine or 4% cocaine can also be used and endoscopy can begin almost at once, since the passage of the endoscope is not painful. Topical anaesthesia of the glottis will be partially achieved by the lidocaine already administered. Further anaesthesia can be obtained by either a crico-thyroid injection or injection of lidocaine through the endoscope. The advantage of a crico-thyroid injection is that the endoscopist can proceed immediately to enter the glottis once seen. The disadvantage is that coughing at the time of injection is sometimes florid. Injection of lidocaine through the suction port requires a skilled assistant. It is wise to practice this beforehand, or use an epidural catheter (end cut off) passed down the suction channel, as a conduit. The injection need not be accurate, 5 ml of 4% lidocaine in the direction of the glottis will be satisfactory. Vision is often lost, but will be restored by asking the patient to take deep breaths.

SEDATION

Few patients should be subjected to a literally awake intubation, and discussion in such terms is alarming to nervous patients. Some sedation is helpful in nearly all cases and the actual intubation can be accompanied by a more-or-less induction dose of intravenous agent. Small increments of midazolam or a propofol infusion are suitable to provide 'conscious sedation'. Sedation should be minimal when there is an element of airway obstruction. This advice needs to be qualified, because in some cases of serious airway obstruction where direct laryngoscopy is certain to be difficult and endoscopy is also difficult because of swelling and secretions, the endoscopist may only have one chance of seeing and entering the glottis. In such dire circumstances it may be necessary to give intravenous anaesthesia and suxamethonium as soon as the endoscope is in the trachea.

POSITION OF PATIENT AND TELEVISION SCREEN

If a television is used it is helpful to position it so that the endoscopist need not turn their head to see it. The position of the endoscopist is generally at the patient's head in anaesthetised patients and beside the patient when the patient is awake. Awake patients feel less threatened if allowed to sit up.

ROTATION

Stiles et al published an account of 100 fibreoptic intubations in 1972. They concluded that the best tubes to use were flexible, reinforced, 'armoured' tubes and it was essential to rotate them constantly as they were passed. This advice is still entirely correct. It is particularly important to use this 'drilling' technique when attempting to pass tubes through the nose or LMA. Failure to rotate is a very common cause of failure. If an armoured tube is not available, it is useful to soften a plastic tube by warming in sterile water. It is foolish to attempt to pass tubes larger than 7.0 mm over a fibreoptic laryngoscope and it is rarely necessary to use a tube larger than 7.0 mm for anaesthesia. Lubricating jelly on the endoscope or tube should be used only at the moment of passing the tube. Jelly on the fingers seriously hampers the operator's ability to manipulate the endoscope and tube. The position of the tube should be checked both endoscopically and by ausculation. It is easy to confuse the carina and the divisions of the right main bronchus.

RETROGRADE FIBREOPTIC INTUBATION

Problems of swelling, distorted anatomy displacing the glottis from the midline and secretions can prevent successful endoscopy. Retrograde fibreoptic intubation can be successful in these situations. A guidewire is introduced into the oral cavity through a crico-thyroid needle; the guidewire is then passed through the endoscope's suction channel (a 2 metre wire is required – a suitable retrograde kit is available from Cook™). The endoscope is advanced until the entry point of the wire into the trachea is seen. The wire is withdrawn through the mouth and the endoscope advanced further into the trachea.

TEACHING FIBREOPTIC INTUBATION

A television system is desirable, and it is difficult to sustain a training programme without one.

It is important to ensure that ventilation of the patient's lungs is not interrupted whilst trainees become familiar with endoscopic appearances. The most satisfactory solution is to place a tracheal tube by direct laryngoscopy in uncomplicated patients. The pupil can then perform endoscopy in an unhurried fashion. The LMA is also useful in instruction, both to allow endoscopic inspection of the glottis via the mask and to facilitate ventilation whilst nasendoscopy is performed. The mask can be removed after nasendoscopy to permit the endoscopist to see the glottis.

KEY POINTS

- Identifying patients that require fibreoptic intubation is sometimes difficult.
- An awake endoscopy should be performed if there is concern regarding ventilation during the procedure.
- Suppression of the cough reflex and sedation is recommended.
- It is important to rotate the tracheal tube over the endoscope during insertion.

FURTHER READING

Caplan RA, Posner KL. Medical-Legal considerations: the ASA closed claims project. In: Benumof JL (ed) Airway management. New York: Mosby, 1996, pp. 944–955

Koh KF, Hare JD, Calder I. Small tubes revisited. Anaesthesia 1998; 53: 46–49

Lechman MJ, Donahoo JS, MacVaugh H III. Endotracheal intubation using percutaneous retrograde guide wire insertion followed by antegrade fiberoptic bronchoscopy. Crit Care Med 1986; 14: 589–590

Ovassapian A. Fiberoptic endoscopy and the difficult airway, 2nd Edn. Philadelphia: Lippincott-Raven, 1996

Shaw IC, Welchew EA, Harrison BJ, Michael S. Complete airway obstruction during awake fibreoptic intubation. Anaesthesia 1997; 52: 576–585

Silk JM, Hill HM, Calder I. Difficult intubation and the laryngeal mask. Eur J Anaesth 1991; 4: 47–51

Smith M, Calder I, Crockard HA, et al. Oxygen saturation and cardiovascular changes during fibreoptic intubation under general anaesthesia. Anaesthesia 1992; 47: 158–161

25

THORACO-LUMBAR SURGERY

C. Williams

INTRODUCTION

Thoraco-lumbar surgery is performed for trauma, congenital anomalies and tumours involving the spine but it is the degenerative diseases (e.g. spondylosis, spondylolisthesis and stenosis) that most commonly lead to spine surgery.

DEGENERATIVE DISEASE

Although spondylosis can occur secondary to trauma, progressive desiccation of the vertebral disc's nucleus pulposus combines with fracture of the surrounding annulus fibrosis to allow the nucleus to herniate, usually at L4/5 or L5/S1 level. Initial pain is due to herniated disc stretching the posterior longitudinal ligament and this is exacerbated by nerve root compression, inflammation and muscle spasm. Urgent surgery is indicated if there are signs of spinal cord compression or a progressively deteriorating neurological examination.

Spondylolisthesis is usually caused by long-standing instability between vertebral bodies, and results in the slipping forward of one vertebral body upon its lower body. It occurs more frequently at L4/5 level particularly in women and the elderly. Posterior lumbar fusion with iliac crest bone grafting or instrumentation is commonly employed to return stability to the joint, which can result in surprising blood loss.

Degenerative spinal stenosis reduces spinal canal volume causing neurogenic claudication. It occurs typically from facet joint hypertrophy or thickening of the ligamentum flavum and in most cases can be surgically decompressed without the need for spinal fusion for stabilisation.

TRAUMA

Trauma can occur anywhere along the spine, particularly the cervical region, and seldom occurs in isolation. However, not all spinal injury requires urgent surgery. Only patients with progressive neurological deficits or where traction fails to relieve compression are operated upon, usually within 24 hours of injury, after full evaluation and resuscitation. The management of spinal cord injury and autonomic hyper-reflexia are outlined in Chapters 35 and 63 respectively.

SCOLIOSIS

Scoliosis can be due to neuromuscular diseases (e.g. muscular dystrophy, poliomyelitis, Friedreich's ataxia or cerebral palsy), mesenchymal conditions (e.g.

Marfan's syndrome, collagen vascular disorders or trauma) or idiopathic. Surgical correction is usually performed when the angle of scoliosis or Cobb angle exceeds 50°, and is directed at relieving thoracic cavity deformity. This deformity can cause restrictive pulmonary disease leading to cor pulmonale. About 25% of patients with idiopathic scoliosis have mitral valve prolapse. Neurological deficits may be present if scoliosis is associated with neural tissue defects.

Scoliosis surgery may compromise spinal cord blood flow and some form of spinal cord monitoring, either an intraoperative wake-up test or somatosensory monitoring (SSEP), or both, are usually performed. Blood loss can also be high and consideration should be given to preoperative autologous blood donation, careful patient positioning, intraoperative hypotension, red cell salvage, or haemodilution techniques. If induced hypotension is employed to decrease blood loss, spinal cord perfusion must never be compromised.

TUMOURS

Spinal cord tumours can be classified as axial (within the cord itself) or extra-axial (alongside the cord). Extra-axial tumours are either intradural or extradural. Wherever the location, tumour resection requires a laminectomy first to achieve adequate access. Spinal cord monitoring, e.g. somatosensory or EMG monitoring, is usually employed in order to preserve neurological function.

GENERAL ANAESTHETIC CONSIDERATIONS

POSITION

Patient position for thoraco-lumbar spine surgery depends upon the chosen surgical approach. Lumbar vertebrectomies are easily performed supine with an anterior approach, whereas a lateral approach is used for thoracic vertebral body surgery with the patient in a severe lateral jackknife position. Most spinal surgery, however, is performed using a posterior approach with the patient prone on a frame or padded rolls to support the chest, leaving the abdomen free. Excessive abdominal pressure compresses the inferior vena cava and distends spinal epidural veins obscuring the surgical field and increasing blood loss. It also limits diaphragmatic excursion leading to dangerous increases in airway pressure. Urine output becomes erratic in prone patients, so central venous and arterial blood pressure monitoring may be required in major cases and should be addressed prior to positioning the patient.

Deep venous thrombosis leading to pulmonary embolus is possible, especially in spinal cord injury patients turned prone.

Venous air embolism is a risk since exposed bone is elevated above the level of the heart when prone. Appropriate precautions should be taken to diagnose and treat its complications. (See Chapter 15)

Pressure applied to an eye can result in retinal injury and ischaemia exacerbated by hypotension or anaemia. Whatever the patient position, adequate padding is needed to protect all pressure points.

ANAESTHETIC TECHNIQUE

A stable anaesthetic is required with particular attention to maintaining spinal cord perfusion. When SSEP monitoring is required, inhalation agents may affect the tracing even at low doses (< 0.5 MAC). Propofol and/or opiate infusion techniques have been reported as being successful in cases that require wake-up testing intraoperatively. Firm securing of the endotracheal tube cannot be overemphasised.

Induced hypotension should be used only if absolutely necessary, and can be achieved with short-acting vasodilators (SNP, GTN) or β-blockers (esmolol, labetalol).

Fluid balance must be maintained. Blood loss can be surprisingly high when performing spinal surgery. Decortication of bone in preparation for fusion, harvesting iliac crest bone for grafting, large incisions for scoliosis repair and resecting metastatic lesions to the spine require particular attention.

Heat loss may be a problem, particularly in scoliosis surgery or other surgery with large incisions and significant blood loss. Intravenous fluids may need to be warmed, and ambient temperature increased. Warming blankets should be used wherever possible.

Intravenous opioids are generally required both intra- and postoperatively. Patient-controlled, or nurse-controlled opioid infusion systems, supplemented with non-steroidal anti-inflammatory drugs, are normally prescribed for postoperative analgesia.

KEY POINTS

- Spinal cord disease may be accompanied by significant systemic disease.
- Management in alternative positions may be needed.
- Blood loss can be substantial.
- Spinal cord monitoring, e.g. wake-up tests or SSEPs, are commonly employed.

FURTHER READING

Hagberg CA, Welch WC, Bowman-Howard ML. Anesthesia and surgery for spine and spinal cord procedures. In: Albin MS (ed.) Textbook of neuroanesthesia: with neurosurgical and neuroscience perspectives. New York: McGraw-Hill, 1997

Mahla ME, Horlocker TT. Vertebral column and spinal cord surgery. In: Cucchiara RF, Black S, Michenfelder JD (eds) Clinical neuroanesthesia, 2nd Edn. New York: Churchill Livingstone, 1998

26

CAROTID ENDARTERECTOMY

A.K. Gupta

INTRODUCTION

Carotid endarterectomy (CEA) has been shown to provide greater benefit than medical treatment in patients presenting with transient ischaemic attacks (TIA) and reversible ischaemic neurologic deficits (RIND) and severe carotid stenosis (70–90% diameter reduction). Recent surveys indicate that CEA is associated with a perioperative mortality between 0.5 and 2%, and morbidity between 2 and 4%. The primary causes of this morbidity and mortality are new neurologic deficits and myocardial infarction.

The three main goals in the perioperative management of CEA are:

1. Haemodynamic stability during induction, maintenance and emergence.
2. Maintenance of adequate cerebral and myocardial perfusion.
3. Rapid emergence to enable early neurological assessment.

PREOPERATIVE MANAGEMENT

Patients are usually hypertensive with some degree of ischaemic heart disease (IHD) for which they are being medically managed. A thorough cardiorespiratory history should be taken with a detailed assessment of the degree of IHD and cerebrovascular disease. Optimisation of medical therapy for all conditions should occur preoperatively, particularly control of hypertension.

Full blood count, electrolytes, coagulation profile, ECG and chest X-ray are regarded as baseline investigations. Echocardiography may be useful in patients with severe IHD and poor exercise tolerance, or those presenting with a new cardiac murmur.

Benzodiazepine premedication is sufficient if required.

ANAESTHETIC TECHNIQUE

Regional Anaesthesia

Regional anaesthesia has been advocated for CEA. Surgery is best performed under a combined deep cervical (C1–4) and superficial cervical plexus block. Minimal or no sedation should be used. The advantage of this method is that awake patients can serve as their own monitor for neurological function. Patients need to be preselected for their ability to cooperate and lie flat and still for the duration of the surgery. Problems arise if surgery is prolonged and if ischaemia occurs during clamping of the ICA. If

deficit does occur then the clamps should be released, the blood pressure elevated and a shunt inserted. Confusion, panic or seizures may be a consequence of ischaemia.

General Anaesthesia

A smooth induction with minimal haemodynamic fluctuations are desirable. The intravenous induction agents have the advantage of reduction in cerebral metabolism which may be protective if ischaemia occurs. Administration of short- or intermediate-acting opiates (fentanyl, alfentanil, remifentanil) contribute towards haemodynamic stability and allow for reduced doses of anaesthetic agents. Short-acting non-depolarising muscle relaxants (atracurium, vecuronium) are appropriate for the duration of surgery.

Maintenance can proceed with nitrous oxide/oxygen supplemented with either 1 MAC inhalation agent (isoflurane or sevoflurane) or a propofol infusion. Hypocapnia should be avoided to prevent cerebral vasoconstriction and hypercapnia may induce a 'steal' phenomenon, therefore normocarbia is recommended.

Heparin 3000–5000 units should be administered intravenously before carotid clamping. During ICA occlusion blood pressure should be maintained at normotension or up to 20% higher than preinduction pressure to ensure adequate cerebral perfusion. This may be achieved by decreasing anaesthetic depth or by the use of an α-agonist either by bolus or infusion. Myocardial ischaemia must be avoided.

Two intraoperative complications may commonly occur:

1. *Bradycardia and hypotension*: This may be due to surgical manipulation of the carotid sinus causing an afferent impulse to the brainstem (CN IX and X) and can be prevented by infiltration of the sinus with local anaesthetic. Occasionally hypertension and tachycardia are observed after clamp application. The variability of response of this reflex may reflect the differing degrees of sinus sensitivity secondary to the atherosclerotic process.
2. *Decreased cerebral perfusion*: This will manifest as a decrease (> 50% reduction) in EEG amplitude and/or mean MCA flow velocity on TCD if monitored. This should be treated by increasing arterial pressure and a bolus of propofol or thiopentone for cerebral protection.

Emergence and extubation is a crucially important period. The aim is to have a patient who awakens rapidly but is haemodynamically stable. As the anaesthetic is reversed, blood pressure begins to rise. If this is not controlled, anastamotic leakage or rupture may occur. Detrimental effects of cerebral hyperaemia may also manifest in the postoperative period. Many of these patients are smokers and have irritable airways and removal of the stimulus of the endotracheal tube after extubation often stabilises blood pressure during emergence. Instillation of 80–100 mg lidocaine into the endotracheal tube or intravenously may reduce coughing and blunt the hypertensive response.

Other pharmacological interventions may be required if hypertension is persistent (> 20% above preoperative pressure). Labetalol, esmolol and nitroprusside are useful drugs at this stage. Nitroglycerine has an added advantage if there is evidence of myocardial ischaemia.

POSTOPERATIVE CONSIDERATIONS

1. *Control of BP*: Hypertension and hypotension need to be prevented. Any deterioration in neurological state needs to be investigated rapidly.
2. *Surgical problems*: Haematoma formation may compromise the airway and needs to be evacuated early. Other surgical complication include paralysis of CNs (VII, IX, X or XII) and carotid body dysfunction.
3. *Cerebrovascular complications*: stroke, emboli, carotid artery thrombosis, hyperperfusion syndrome.
4. *Myocardial infarction*.

Monitoring

In addition to routine intraoperative monitoring, invasive arterial BP monitoring is regarded as mandatory. Central venous lines or pulmonary artery catheters may be inserted if clinically indicated.

Several methods of monitoring cerebral perfusion intraoperatively may be used:

1. *Middle cerebral artery flow velocity (MCAFvx)*: This is measured with transcranial Doppler ultrasonography (TCD) by insonating the MCA. Greater than 50% reduction in MCAFvx and EEG has been shown to be predictive of ischaemia and a shunt should be placed.

2. *EEG*: Reduction in EEG (or SSEP) activity are considered indicative of potentially serious ischaemia.
3. *NIRS*: Changes in concentrations of oxygenated and deoxygenated haemoglobin measured by NIRS may help in assessing regional cerebral ischaemia.
4. *Stump pressure*: This is a measure of pressure of the carotid stump distal to the occluded artery. Poor perfusion is generally taken as a stump pressure <50 mmHg. However stump pressures >50 mmHg do not ensure adequate regional perfusion.

A more detailed description of these monitors are given in their individual chapters.

KEY POINTS

- Patients presenting for CEA are at increased risk of perioperative morbidity and mortality.
- CEA can be performed under regional or general anaesthesia.
- Maintenance of haemodynamic stability and adequate cerebral perfusion is required.
- Appropriate monitoring is required to prevent cerebral ischaemia.
- Tight blood pressure control is important during the recovery period.

FURTHER READING

North American Symptomatic Carotid Endarterectomy Trial Collaborators: Beneficial effect of carotid endarterectomy in symptomatic patients with high grade carotid stenosis. N Engl J Med 1991; 325: 445–453

European Carotid Surgery Trialists' Collaborative Group. MRC European Carotid Surgery Trial. Interim results for symptomatic patients with severe (70–99%) or with mild (0–29%) carotid stenosis. Lancet 1991; 337: 1235–1243

Kirkpatrick PJ, Lam J, Al-Rawi P, Smielewski P, Czosnyka M. Defining thresholds for critical ischaemia by using near-infrared spectroscopy in the adult brain. J Neurosurg 1998; 89: 389–394

Erwin D, Pick MJ, Taylor GW. Anaesthesia for carotid surgery. Anaesthesia 1980; 35: 246

27

ANAESTHESIA FOR INTERVENTIONAL NEURORADIOLOGY

J. M. Turner

INTRODUCTION

Interventional neuroradiology is growing quickly, as better imaging equipment and new materials become available to the radiologist. Anaesthesia must develop to accommodate the new techniques and, as radiological procedures are associated with a significant morbidity, a careful audit of results is particularly necessary in the period of rapid growth to define the ultimate usefulness of interventional radiology.

GENERAL PROBLEMS OF ANAESTHESIA IN X-RAY

HOSTILE ENVIRONMENT

Anaesthetists need to know how to protect themselves from ionising radiation. A lead apron with a 0.35 mm lead equivalent must be worn and close exposure to the radiation source avoided. The room must be organised so that the anaesthetist can see the airway, anaesthetic machine, lung ventilator and vital signs monitor from behind a lead glass screen.

MOVEMENT

The X-ray couch on which the patient lies will be moved by the radiologist during the examination to allow screening of different body areas. In neuroradiology, the movement may extend from screening of the abdomen as the vascular catheter is passed up the aorta to screening of the head. The breathing tubes, monitoring cables and infusion lines must be arranged and fixed and long enough to be tolerant of such movement.

EQUIPMENT

The gantry carrying the X-ray tube is often big and bulky. Nevertheless it needs to move around the patient's head to image the cerebral circulation in many projections. The placing of monitoring cables and lines must be arranged so that they are out of the X-ray field and do not impede the rapid movement of the X-ray tube gantry. Interventional procedures may be quite prolonged and if the radiographer is able to move the X-ray tube quickly, without it catching on monitoring cable or lines, then the procedure will not be further prolonged.

STAFF

The X-ray Department is not an operating theatre and staff working there may not be familiar with anaesthetic routines. New procedures in neuroradiology may be high-risk procedures and it is important to train the technical and nursing staff so that they are familiar with the risks of anaesthesia and therefore able to help the anaesthetist.

ANAESTHETIC DRUGS AND TECHNIQUES

Anaesthetic drugs that have an effect on the cerebral circulation, whether directly, or indirectly by affecting cerebral metabolism, may alter radiographic appearances. The vasodilation produced by some anaesthetic agents may mean that the angiographic images are less clear, because the bolus of contrast cannot fill the vascular lumen. Conversely, vasoconstriction, such as that produced by hyperventilation, not only improves the quality of the images, but also allows more images to be taken because the cerebral circulation is slowed.

INTERVENTIONAL NEURORADIOLOGY

Interventional neuroradiology is most commonly used for obliterating an aneurysm, for treating an arteriovenous malformation or for reducing the blood flow to a vascular tumour before surgery. In most cases, a large vascular sheath (7.5 F) is placed in the femoral artery and a catheter passed through the sheath to one of the major cerebral vessels. Finer catheters and guidewires are passed through this catheter into the cerebral vessels and up to the lesion. Angiography is performed at all stages of the procedure to delineate the anatomy. The X-ray image is processed to subtract out radio-opaque structures such as bone, so that the vascular anatomy is clearer. A 'road map' image is available, where an angiogram view is retained on the radiologist's monitor screen with the current screening view superimposed on top.

ANEURYSM

The treatment of intracerebral aneurysms has been advanced by the development of the Guglielmi detachable coils,[1] which are platinum coils attached to a stainless steel guidewire. The coil is passed through a fine catheter and in the aneurysmal sac opens to hold itself in position. Angiography is performed to check that the position of the coil is satisfactory. The connection between the guidewire and coil is fused by passing an electrical current through the system. The guidewire is then removed, leaving the coil in place. Several coils may be required for an aneurysm.

ARTERIOVENOUS MALFORMATIONS

This condition presents a dramatic picture on angiography, with many feeding vessels and large, arterialised draining veins produced by the fistulae. Flow through the AVM is extremely rapid and not under autoregulatory control. Embolisation is frequently performed in several stages and in some centres conscious sedation is preferred.[2] The main advantage of conscious sedation is that when a microcatheter is placed ready for the embolisation, the safety of the placement can be checked by injection of sodium amytal (30 mg) or lignocaine (30 mg) with subsequent neurological assessment.[3] General anaesthesia does not easily allow for such an examination, but does allow the manipulation of the $PaCO_2$ as well as the production of hypo- or hypertension as required. Many materials have been used for embolisation, including contact adhesive (N–butyl–cyanoacrylate), coils and pellets of silastic. More recently the use of an ethylene vinyl alcohol co-polymer in dimethyl sulphoxide (DMSO) solvent has been recommended.

The successful placement of the embolic material within the AVM, avoiding it passing through to the venous circulation, may be quite difficult and the ability of the anaesthetist to modify blood flow to the AVM is valuable. Many techniques can be used, but we use a combination of hypotension, produced by labetalol and sodium nitroprusside.[4] Once a stable level of hypotension has been produced, Positive End-Expired Pressure (PEEP) is applied to the airway as the radiologist injects the embolic material, temporarily to reduce venous outflow.

MONITORING

Full monitoring, with oximetry, direct intra-arterial and central venous pressures and ECG is essential. Cerebral function may be monitored clinically if the patient is under conscious sedation. Anticoagulation is required and should be closely monitored with hourly measurements of APTT and PT.

COMPLICATIONS

Neuroradiology has a significant morbidity.[5] The two most serious complications of interventional radiology are haemorrhage and vascular occlusion. Haemorrhage takes place into the intact skull, so cardiovascular disturbance is noticeable. Control of any undue hypertension with thiopentone or propofol will help to minimise the extent of the intracranial bleeding. In their study, Young and Pile-Spellman are insistent on the necessity for the immediate reversal of the heparinisation.[3]

Vascular occlusion may lead to cerebral infarction if it is untreated. It may be due to thrombosis, or the malpositioning of catheters, coils, or other embolic material. Vascular spasm may also be induced and may be treated by phentolamine. Thrombolysis may be required. Induced hypertension may be indicated to maintain cerebral perfusion.

KEY POINTS

- Interventional neuroradiology is growing fast, requiring careful audit
- Anaesthesia in the X-ray Department has special problems
- Great care must be taken to maintain safety for the patient
- The anaesthetist can manipulate the cerebral circulation to aid the radiologist

REFERENCES

1. Guglielmi G, Vinuela F, Duckwiler G et al. Endovascular treatment of posterior circulation aneurysms by electrothrombosis using electrically detachable coils. J Neurosurg 1992; 77: 515–524
2. Menon DK, Gupta AK. Anaesthesia and sedation for diagnostic procedures. Curr Opin Anesthiol 1994; 7: 495–499
3. Young WL, Pile-Spellman J. Anesthetic considerations for interventional neuroradiology. Anesthesiology 1994; 80: 427–456
4. O'Mahony BJ, Bolsin SNC. Anaesthesia for closed embolisation of cerebral arterial malformations. Anaesth Intensive Care 1988; 16: 318–323
5. Purdy PD, Batjer HH, Samson D. Management of hemorrhagic complications from preoperative embolization of arteriovenous malformations. J Neurosurg 1991; 3: 101–106

28

ANAESTHESIA AND SEDATION FOR MAGNETIC RESONANCE IMAGING

D.K. Menon

INTRODUCTION

Magnetic field strengths in use for MRI are measured in units termed Tesla (T). One Tesla equals 10 000 Gauss (G). The magnetic field strength at the surface of the earth is of the order of 0.5–1.5 G. Field strengths used in MRI range from 0.05 to 2.0 T. Higher strengths are associated with better spatial resolution and tend to be based on cryogenic magnets with superconducting coils operating in liquid helium.

MRI SAFETY ISSUES

PROJECTILE RISKS FROM FERROMAGNETIC OBJECTS AND EFFECTS ON FERROMAGNETIC IMPLANTS

Oxygen cylinders, identification badges, scissors and paging devices carried in by clinical staff constitute common risks to patients, and all individuals entering the MRI suite should be screened for such objects, which should be left outside the suite. Ferromagnetic objects that must be in the vicinity of the MRI suite (such as oxygen cylinders) should be stationed outside the 50 G line.

While many implanted clinical devices are non-ferromagnetic, movement of implanted ferromagnetic objects under the influence of the magnet can be catastrophic. While categorised lists of implants exist, manufacturers have been known to change the composition of objects without notification. Some implanted ferromagnetic objects are safe, either because they are too small or they are firmly anchored in place by the surrounding tissue, for example surgical clips that have been in-situ for years. Most units have a comprehensive checklist for patients to complete prior to entering the scanning suite. Metal detectors are too insensitive to play any role in screening patients prior to MR examinations. Screening for intraocular foreign objects has caused controversy, since movement of a metal foreign body in the eye can cause vitreous haemorrhage and loss of the eye. If a patient has no symptoms and a series of plain radiographs of the orbits does not demonstrate a radiopaque foreign body, most centres would agree that an MR scan can be performed safely.

While product information supplied with aneurysm clips will make statements regarding MR compatibility or otherwise, repeated handling and sterilisation could induce ferromagnetism in some previously non-magnetic alloys. It has been concluded by some authorities that only one of two criteria permit completely safe MR studies in a patient who has an intracranial aneurysm clip: a previous uneventful MR scanning *at the same field strength*, or the implant having been tested with a powerful hand held magnet prior to application by the neurosurgeon. Web sites on the Internet provide useful information regarding a large range of other implants and devices. These are listed in Table 28.1.

NON-FERROMAGNETIC OBJECTS AND IMPLANTS

These must also be treated with caution as they can distort or degrade the quality of the image, and the application of oscillating radiofrequency (RF) fields can lead to heating and burns from any metallic equipment or implant. Burns are the most common injury to patients associated with MRI, and result when a conductive loop is created between the patient's skin and a conductor, such as electrocardiographic leads or pulse oximeter probes. The risk of burns may be minimised by ensuring that insulation on wires is intact and separating them from skin with padding, avoiding large loops of wire that lead to the induction of currents, and applying sensors as far away from the imaged area as possible.

When patients have metallic implants it is standard practice to ask them to indicate if the area in question feels warm or uncomfortable. This is not possible in the anaesthetised patient. An assessment of risk should be obtained from the radiological staff in the MRI unit prior to the scan and the patient warned accordingly. Such potential sites must also be checked for evidence of injury at the end of the procedure.

Table 28.1 Useful Internet sites for information regarding MR safety	
Federal Drug Agency, USA	http://www.fda.gov/cdrh/ode/primerf6.html
UK Medical Devices Agency	http://www.medical-devices.gov.uk/
International MR Safety Central Web Site	http://kanal.arad.upmc.edu/mrsafety.html

IMPLANTED ELECTRICALLY, MAGNETICALLY AND MECHANICALLY ACTIVATED DEVICES

MRI may interfere with the operation of such devices, or result in image distortion or burns. Cardiac pacemakers are the most common electrically activated devices found in patients referred for MRI. The acceptable safe level for exposure to magnetic fringe fields for patients with cardiac pacemakers are currently set at 5 G. At fields above this the pacemaker will go into fixed rate mode, and may trigger ventricular fibrillation. In essence, MRI is contraindicated in any person who has any implanted device, unless it is known for absolute certainty that the device will function safely.

POTENTIAL BIOLOGICAL EFFECTS

Higher strength magnetic fields and rapidly switched gradient fields can cause sensations of altered taste, dizziness and nausea. Exposure to gradient or radiofrequency fields experienced by scanned subjects can reach biologically relevant levels and produce local heating effects as described above. This exposure is clearly regulated by bodies such as the Federal Drug Agency (FDA) in the USA and the National Radiological Protection Board (NRPB) in the UK. While available human data generally supports the safety of exposure to low magnetic fields in clinical staff, there is currently an impetus to measure occupational exposure to static, gradient and radiofrequency fields and define safe limits for exposure.

OTHER ISSUES

The contrast agent, gadopentate dimeglumine (Gd-DTPA, Magnevist®) can improve image quality and has an excellent safety record in comparison to other contrast agents, with only one reported fatality from anaphylaxis. Cryogenic magnets with superconducting coils operate in liquid helium that boils (quenches) rapidly if the cryostat temperature rises. The released helium dilutes room oxygen and the cold vapour causes frostbite and cryogenic burns.

MONITORING DURING MRI

MRI demands an immobile patient be placed in a noisy, dark, cold and uncomfortable space and isolated from radiology and anaesthetic staff. Anaesthesia or sedation may be required in paediatric or uncooperative subjects, or in critically ill patients. The FDA in the USA, http://www.fda.gov/cdrh/ode/primerf6.html, has provided useful definitions against which the performance of clinical equipment can be assessed in an MR environment. The terms *MR safe* and *MR compatible* are used to define equipment properties so that their use within an MR environment can be ascertained. The term *MR safe* indicates that when a device is used in the MR suite it presents no additional risk to the patient; while the term *MR compatible* indicates that a device is both *MR safe* **and** has been demonstrated to neither significantly affect the diagnostic quality of the imaging procedure, nor have its operations affected by the MR scanning system. In practice, many monitoring and infusion devices function normally at fields of 50 G or less, but may be neither MR safe (since they present a projectile risk due to ferromagnetic components) nor MR compatible, since stray RF interference from the device may make imaging impossible. Devices such as colour cathode ray screens may be distorted in fields exceeding 1–2 G, while monochrome screens function reasonably well up to 5 G. Liquid crystal display screens are not distorted at all. Magnetic tape and computer discs are corrupted in fields greater than 30 G.

The ECG shows significant changes within a static magnetic field. Leads I, II, V1 and V2 are the worst affected, with changes in early T waves and late ST segments mimicking hyperkalaemia or pericarditis. The radiofrequency currents used during MRI also produce artefacts of the ECG from current induction in ECG cables. ECG output during MRI can be improved by filtering or gating, the use of shielded or carbon fibre cables, telemetry or fibreoptic systems. Patients have received burns from conventional pulse oximeter probes. Pulse oximetry systems based on fibreoptic technology are now available; these devices operate without interference during MRI and are safe. While long sampling lines have been used for respiratory gas monitoring, very long tubing can increase resistance and lag times to detect disconnection. The availability of MR compatible gas monitors has made the use of such long sampling tubes unnecessary.

Invasive blood pressure monitoring can be measured accurately, as can ICP via a ventriculostomy. Parenchymal ICP sensors present more of a problem, but there are early reports of the safe use of a Codman microtransducer, monitored through a fibreoptic link. Both peripheral and central core temperatures can be measured accurately using probes incorporating radiofrequency filters.

INTEGRATED MONITORING UNITS

In the past many departments have adapted existing equipment to form satisfactory integrated monitoring systems. The availability of commercial systems for safe monitoring makes such home made solutions completely unacceptable (Table 28.2). A typical MR system costs in excess of one million pounds, and there seems little justification to avoid spending £30,000 to ensure safe anaesthesia in this context.

SEDATION AND ANAESTHESIA FOR MRI

PREANAESTHETIC PREPARATION

It is essential to determine contraindications to MRI prior to induction of anaesthesia. The anaesthetist must also ensure that they are familiar with the MR installation, particularly the extent of fringe fields and the location of resuscitation equipment. The use of earplugs or other auditory protection can substantially reduce the stimulation associated with imaging, and permit the use of lower doses of sedatives or anaesthetic agents. Anaesthetic equipment may be positioned within the MRI suite, or outside it. The former solution will mean that the anaesthetist will be unable to leave the room without interrupting the scan, the latter will limit access to the patient to interscan intervals, except in an emergency

CONDUCT OF ANAESTHESIA

Induction of anaesthesia should ideally take place outside the 50 G line with dedicated equipment. Standard Macintosh laryngoscopes are not ferromagnetic but do undergo a degree of torque in a strong magnetic field. Standard laryngoscope batteries are highly magnetic. Fibreoptic light sources or plastic laryngoscopes powered by paper- or plastic-jacketed lithium batteries are available. Standard hospital trolleys are highly ferromagnetic and special trolleys should be available for use in the MRI suite.

While sedation is commonly used, particularly in children, it must be undertaken with care. Techniques employed for sedation of children include ketamine, barbiturates, benzodiazepines, high dose chloral hydrate (50–150 mg/kg) and low dose propofol infusions. Sedation can only be safely employed for MRI in children provided they are accompanied by trained personnel and are adequately monitored. Supplementary oxygen should be given to all patients.

Laryngeal mask airways (LMA) reinforced with a metal spiral are ferromagnetic and produce substantial imaging artefacts; however, newer reinforced LMAs containing plastic spirals can be used during MR studies. When intubation is undertaken, use of a preformed endotracheal tube is preferable. After the head coils are in place there may be little room for anything protruding from the mouth. Unless there is a specific indication, it is not absolutely necessary to ventilate patients for MRI. Both inhalational anaesthesia using halothane or isoflurane, and total intravenous anaesthesia with propofol, have been used successfully for spontaneously breathing and ventilated patients. A suitable recovery area, equipped with monitoring equipment, suction apparatus, oxygen and trained staff should be located outside the 50 G line.

Although a number of infusion devices do function accurately, most are ferromagnetic, malfunction or are inaccurate in fringe fields. Pumps must be supported on non-ferromagnetic poles. Needles and intravenous cannulae are usually non-ferromagnetic but should be tested before use. The surface of trolleys used for MRI is very firm and should be suitably padded to prevent the development of pressure sores, especially in critically ill patients.

STRATEGIC ISSUES

Perhaps the most common continuing problems in connection with anaesthesia in the MRI environment pertain to a lack of strategic thinking when such facilities are being constructed. The provision of filtered AC power, piped anaesthetic gases and ports in the RF shield costs relatively little at the time of

Table 28.2 *Representative* list of manufacturers of MRI compatible equipment		
Monitoring	MR Equipment Corporation, USA	www.mrequipment.com
	Bruker Gmbh, Germany	www.bruker.de/
	Masimo Corporation, USA	www.masimo.com
Anaesthetic equipment	Datex-Ohmeda	www.datex-ohmeda.com
	North American Drager, USA	www.nad.com
Ventilators	Sims Pneupac	www.pneupac.com
Infusion pumps	Mammendorfer Institut für Physik und Medezin, Germany	www.mipm.com

initial construction. It is equally important that a realistic assessment be made of needs for anaesthesia and supervised sedation during scans, and resources be identified (both in terms of money and people) to meet these needs.

KEY POINTS

- Sedation and anaesthesia are likely to be increasingly required for MRI examinations in specific patient groups.
- The commercial availability of MRI compatible monitoring and anaesthetic equipment allows safe clinical practice without compromises.
- It is important that strategic decisions regarding anaesthetic utilities be addressed when new MRI suites are being built.
- Careful attention to detail and preparation to MRI safety issues are important before embarking on anaesthesia for individual patients.

- Safe anaesthesia in an MRI environment depends on well designed protocols and systems, not just on individual competence and care.

RECOMMENDED READING

Menon DK, Gupta AK. 1994 Anaesthesia and sedation for diagnostic procedures. *Current Opinion in Anaesthesiology* 7, 495–499.

Menon DK, Peden CJ, Hall AS, Sargentoni J, Whitwam JG. 1992 Magnetic resonance for the anaesthetist. Part I: physical principles, applications, safety aspects. *Anaesthesia* 47, 240–255.

Peden CJ, Menon DK, Hall AS, Sargentoni J, Whitwam JG. 1992 Magnetic resonance for the anaesthetist. Part 2: anaesthesia and monitoring in MR units. *Anaesthesia* 47, 508–517.

Shellock FG, Kanal E. 1994 *Magnetic Resonance. Bioeffects, Safety and Patient Management.* New York: Raven Press.

29

SHUNT SURGERY

A. Summors

INTRODUCTION

Hydrocephalus is usually due to obstruction of CSF flow giving rise to increases in volume and consequently intracranial pressure. Surgical insertion of a shunt enables drainage of CSF from the ventricular system into a distal site. The most common drainage site is to the peritoneal cavity but the right atrium, cisterna magna and pleural cavity are also sometimes used.

EQUIPMENT AND SURGICAL PROCEDURE

Shunt systems usually involve three components: a ventricular catheter, a one-way valve and a distal catheter. Other devices may also be incorporated, e.g. on–off valves, siphon control devices and chambers for flushing the shunt system.

The ventricular catheter is inserted through a burr hole connected to the one-way valve which determines the draining pressure from the ventricle, which is then connected to the peritoneal catheter. This is passed subcutaneously from the scalp incision over the occipitoparietal region, over the chest wall to the abdominal incision made either in the midline above the umbilicus or just lateral to and above the umbilicus. The tubing is inserted into the peritoneal cavity through a small abdominal incision. Intravenous antibiotics may be given perioperatively.[1]

PATIENT POSITION

For ventriculo-peritoneal (V-P) shunts, the child is placed supine with the head turned to the opposite side allowing occipital insertion of the ventricular catheter. A towel is placed under the nape of the neck in children or ipsilateral shoulder in adults in order to align the head, neck and abdomen in one plane, allowing easier passage of the subcutaneous tunnelling device for shunt placement.

ANAESTHETIC MANAGEMENT

The patient presenting for insertion of V-P shunt or shunt revision must be considered to have raised ICP. Patients may be neurologically obtunded preoperatively and premedication is often not required.

The anaesthetic technique requires a smooth induction, preferably with an intravenous induction agent using thiopentone or propofol. As many of these patients are children, attempts at intravenous cannulation prior to induction may be distressing which will further increase ICP. In these circumstances an inhalation induction is acceptable.

Patients should be paralysed with a short-acting non-depolarising muscle relaxant prior to intubation. The pressor responses and ICP changes to laryngoscopy and intubation can be limited by a bolus of lignocaine or intravenous agent just prior to intubation. This, however, seems less of a problem in children with open sutures than in adults. After intubation the breathing circuit is secured firmly preventing dragging on the endotracheal tube and the eyes and limbs are protected from injury.

Anaesthesia can be maintained with either a total intravenous technique using propofol, or with a volatile agent. Analgesia is required to cover the initial skin incision and burr hole and the tunnelling of the drain to the abdomen. Fentanyl (1–3 μg/kg) is usually sufficient.

Mild hypocapnia helps reduce ICP and surgical infiltration with 1% lidocaine and epinephrine helps reduce scalp bleeding and provides analgesia.[2] Profound haemodynamic changes may occur if a large volume of CSF is drained rapidly when the ventricular catheter is inserted.

Care must be taken when using the rigid tunnelling device as this theoretically reduces chest wall compliance and may cause either underventilation during pressure controlled ventilation or dangerous increases in airway pressures when volume controlled ventilation is used.

At the conclusion of surgery, patients should be extubated. Any focal neurological signs postoperatively should prompt an urgent CT scan to exclude an intracranial haematoma.

KEY POINTS

- V-P shunts are a common neurosurgical procedure frequently performed in children.
- Patients usually have raised ICP.
- A smooth induction is required.
- Tunnelling the shunt to the abdomen is highly stimulating.
- Patients should have improved neurology postoperatively.

REFERENCES

1. Roth PA, Cohen AR. Management of hydrocephalus in children. In: Tindall GT, Cooper PR, Barrow PL

(eds) The practice of neurosurgery. Baltimore: Williams & Wilkins, 1996, pp. 2707–2728

2. Abou-Madi MN, Trop D, Barnes J. Aetiology and control of cardiovascular reactions during transsphenoidal resection of pituitary microadenomas. Can Anes Soc J 1980; 27: 491–495

FURTHER READING

Messick Jr JM, Newberg LA, Nugent M, Faust RJ. Principles of neuroanesthesia for the neurosurgical patient with CNS pathophysiology. Anesth Analg 1985; 64: 143–174

30

ANAESTHESIA FOR PAEDIATRIC NEUROSURGERY

J.M. Turner

INTRODUCTION

The child requiring neurosurgery presents all the general problems of paediatric anaesthesia, but in addition there are specific problems related to the neurosurgical condition. The spectrum of neurosurgical disease in childhood is different from that in the adult. There are major differences in cerebral physiology. The brain represents 10–15% of the body weight at term and doubles in weight by 6 months of age. The skull is not completely closed, the anterior fontanelle remaining open until 15-18 months. CBF and cerebral metabolic rate ($CMRO_2$) are relatively higher than in the adult.[1] The major neurosurgical problems can be broadly divided by age group:

The premature child and the infant:

1. Ventricular drainage
2. Shunt surgery
3. Third Ventriculostomy
4. Myelomeningocoele
5. Vein of Galen aneurysm.

The child from 2 to 7 years:

1. Diagnostic procedures
2. Space-occupying lesions
3. Trauma
4. AVM.

THE PREMATURE CHILD AND THE INFANT

The management of CSF obstruction and CSF drainage systems requires careful surgery and attention to detail. Shunt surgery is still affected by a high complication rate including infection, shunt blockage and over drainage of CSF.

The premature infant is prone to intraventricular haemorrhage and therefore CSF obstruction. Initially this may be managed by an external ventricular drain, or by the subcutaneous implantation of a reservoir such as an Ommaya reservoir. The complete shunt system of ventricular catheter, valve and drainage tube either to the peritoneum or right atrium is inserted when the high CSF protein resulting from the intraventricular haemorrhage has fallen to normal levels.

On occasions CSF drainage can be improved by an anterior third ventriculostomy, where a communication is produced directly between the third ventricle and the basal cisterns by an endoscopic approach.

The child presenting for surgery to relieve CSF obstruction must be considered to have raised ICP. This is easily confirmed by palpation of the anterior fontanelle and noting whether it is tense, or frankly bulging. Vomiting, caused by the raised ICP may well produce dehydration and electrolyte imbalance. Induction and maintenance of anaesthesia should therefore take into account the raised ICP. The fact that the fontanelles are open and the sutures unfused does not protect the child against high ICP, and as in neuroanaesthesia in the adult all anaesthetic techniques and agents causing an increase in ICP should be avoided.

The well recognised difficulties surrounding intubation of the trachea in the neonate are further complicated if the large head produced by hydrocephalus results in flexion of the neck. If so, a support under the thorax may be required to produce optimal conditions for intubation. A large head may produce a misleading weight in a small infant.

MYELOMENINGOCOELE AND ENCEPHALOCOELE

Disorders of development affecting the neuraxis may produce encephalocoele and myelomeningocoele. Such a defect needs to be closed quickly after delivery, so that neurological deterioration is limited. All the problems of anaesthesia in the neonatal period therefore apply. In addition, the neonate will have to be positioned prone. The myelomeningocoele needs to be protected from damage so, during induction, the neonate may need to be tilted to one side, or if supine, supported on pads leaving the mengiomyelocoele free. The surgeon may need to use a nerve stimulator, so monitoring the degree of neuromuscular block may be helpful (see Chapter 32).

PREMATURE FUSION OF CRANIAL SUTURES

Many syndromes may arise, depending on which cranial suture, or sutures are involved. The skull base and facial sutures may also be affected. High ICP may result, depending on how early the abnormal skull shape is recognised.

Surgery involves cutting the fused suture; the skin incision is extensive and blood loss may therefore be significant.

ANEURYSM OF THE VEIN OF GALEN

Aneurysms of the vein of Galen classically present during the neonatal period with cardiac failure. Late presentation does occur, when the signs may be those of space-occupation or peri-orbital venous congestion. Successful treatment is difficult.

THE CHILD FROM 2 TO 7 YEARS

Space-occupying lesions (SOL) and head trauma are more frequent in this age group. Indeed, intracranial tumours are the second most common neoplasms occuring in childhood. About 70% of SOL are situated in the posterior fossa. Some arteriovenous malformations present in childhood, but large AVMs are rare.[2] Anaesthesia may be required for imaging techniques (angiography and CT or MRI scanning); sedation for such procedures is often unreliable.

As in the adult, the extent of intracranial space-occupation needs to be assessed as well as the degree of oedema formation and whether or not CSF obstruction is present. The likely vascularity of the SOL must be considered, taking into account the probable histology.

GENERAL COMMENTS ON ANAESTHESIA

The principles of good paediatric anaesthesia and good neuroanaesthesia must be applied. The scalp is very vascular and significant blood loss may occur, though good surgical technique should reduce this loss to a minimum. The head is covered by surgical drapes and therefore the care of the airway must be faultless. The flexibility of the neck in children and the awkward position frequently required for neurosurgery means that an armoured endotracheal tube should be used and carefully fixed. Armoured tracheal tubes are available with a Murphy eye, down to the smallest sizes. In the neonate, the tip of the endotracheal tube moves an average of 14.4 mm when the head and neck are moved from full flexion to full extension[3] so auscultation of the chest must be performed after positioning. Fixation of the tube must not obstruct cerebral venous drainage.

Intravenous induction using thiopentone or propofol is valuable, especially where raised ICP exists. Sevoflurane is a valuable alternative as its effects on ICP are minimal[4] and induction is rapid and smooth. Muscle relaxation is indicated and pressure ventilation should be adjusted to produce mild hyperventilation. The use of PEEP must be carefully monitored to ensure that ICP is not adversely affected. If hand ventilation is employed it is important that the airway pressure should be measured so as to ensure effective ventilation without raising ICP. The same agents may effectively be used for the maintenance of anaesthesia.

Maintenance of temperature may be difficult. The exposure of the head promotes cooling. In shunt surgery the need to expose head, chest and abdomen means that warming blankets covering the child cannot be used. The child should therefore lie on a heated mattress and warm air using tubes around the child but under the surgical drapes are valuable. With such problems, accurate temperature measurement is particularly important.

Monitoring should be comprehensive. All patients require oximetry, blood pressure, ECG and end-tidal CO_2. Children with space-occupying lesions require direct intra-arterial monitoring of arterial pressure and if the tumour is vascular, central venous pressure measurements are of value. Estimation of blood loss may be difficult, because a common practice is to moisten the surgical swabs, so that swab weighing gives an inaccurate estimate of blood loss. Oesophageal measurements of temperature are reliable and an oesophageal stethoscope is often recommended.

POSTOPERATIVE CARE

Postoperatively the child should be nursed in a specialised recovery or intensive care unit. The premature infant and the neonate may benefit from a period of controlled ventilation as may children with tumours in the posterior fossa. Otherwise a full recovery allows good monitoring of cerebral function.

KEY POINTS

- There are differences in the cerebral physiology between adults and children.
- The major neurosurgical problems can be broadly divided by age group.
- Anaesthetic management combines the principles of paediatric anaesthesia and neuroanaesthesia.
- Estimation of fluid balance may be difficult particularly after mannitol therapy or blood loss.
- A short period of postoperative ventilation is often required in the premature infant.

REFERENCES

1. Ogawa A, Sakurai Y, Kayama K. 1989 Regional cerebral blood flow with age: changes in cerebral blood flow in childhood. *Neurological Research* 11, 173.
2. Millar C, Bissonnette B, Humphreys RP. 1994 Cerebral arteriovenous malformations in children. *Canadian Journal of Anaesthesia* 41, 321–331.
3. Todres ID, De Bros F, Kramer SS, Moylan FMB, Shannon DS. 1976 Endotracheal displacement in the newborn infant. *Journal of Paediatrics* 89, 126.
4. Takahashi H, Murata K, Ikeda K. 1993 Sevoflurane does not increase intracranial pressure in hyperventilated dogs. *British Journal of Anaesthesia* 71, 551–555.

31

CONGENITAL CRANIOFACIAL PROCEDURES

J. Shapiro

INTRODUCTION

Craniofacial anomalies are frequently a part of a number of common as well as uncommon syndromes. The prevalence is difficult to determine because of the number of syndromes in which they present. These structural defects may be due to fetal developmental anomalies or premature fusion of one or more of the cranial sutures following birth (craniosynostosis).

CLINICAL PROBLEMS

INCREASED ICP

Most of the infants with craniofacial anomalies will have some degree of increased ICP. This may be most pronounced in infants with premature closure of major suture lines.

DIFFICULT AIRWAY ACCESS

Difficulty in laryngoscopic visualisation of the glottic structures varies with the syndrome. Isolated cranial vault anomalies do not usually present with airway difficulties. However, many of the congenital syndromes which have major facial involvement (e.g. Pierre-Robin, Goldenhar) can present as significant intubation challenges.

BLOOD LOSS

Significant blood loss may be expected in any of the surgical repairs for craniofacial anomalies. Procedures involving reshaping of the cranial vault and/or forehead and upper face, in particular, may result in losses of one-third to one-half of the patient's estimated blood volume.

ANAESTHETIC MANAGEMENT

ASSESSMENT AND PREMEDICATION

A survey of other organ systems, principally the cardiovascular and renal systems, should be made to assess for other significant congenital defects. A history of nausea, vomiting, or ataxia suggests significant ICP. A careful assessment of the upper airway including the relative size of the mandible, tongue and oral opening should be made. Evaluation of possible venous and arterial access may suggest the need to have special paediatric central line equipment available prior to induction.

Infants under 6 months of age should not require preoperative medication. The use of premedication in the older infant or toddler should be considered to facilitate smooth induction and decrease agitation which may increase ICP with crying and breath-holding. However, the over-sedated infant may have decreased respiratory effort and increases in ICP secondary to hypercarbia. Oral midazolam (0.5–0.7 mg/kg – max. dose 10 mg) can be very effective in these patients if intravenous access is not available prior to induction.

CONDUCT OF ANAESTHESIA

Most of these patients will arrive in the operating theatre with no i.v. access and inhalational induction is often the method of choice. Prior to induction, minimal monitoring should include pulse oximetry and a precordial stethoscope. As the inhalation induction proceeds (usually with sevoflurane or halothane in oxygen/nitrous oxide) an assistant should place additional monitors, as tolerated, including ECG, non-invasive BP cuff, and temperature probe. If ICP concerns exist, the patient should be moderately hyperventilated. Intravenous access should be obtained with a large-bore cannula as is reasonable based on the patient's size. Note that the saphenous vein is usually quite large and a 22 g or larger cannula can usually be placed for later volume resuscitation even in infants. If not previously obtained, a sample should be sent to the blood bank for cross-match of two 'adult' units of packed red cells. Following securing of the airway with an endotracheal tube, a second i.v. should be obtained as well as arterial access for continuous monitoring of BP. At the time of skin incision, mannitol (1 g/kg) is administered. A brisk diuresis usually ensues shortly after administration and it is important to closely monitor haemodynamic parameters to maintain adequate intravascular volume. Once the craniectomies are started, furosemide (0.5–1 mg/kg) may be administered if the dura looks 'tight', but this is rarely required after mannitol administration. If subcutaneous/intradermal local anaesthetic solutions are utilised by the surgeons prior to incision, opiate requirements are reduced.

Continuous assessment of blood loss is required, keeping in mind that most of the blood lost will be hidden in the surgical drapes. Most patients will require replacement with red blood cells. It is best to wait until the haemoglobin drops to about 8 g/dl before transfusing unless the infant has heart disease or other co-existing pathology requiring a greater oxygen carrying capacity. At that point, a continuous transfusion totalling 20–25 ml/kg over the remaining course of the procedure will usually increase the haemoglobin to 12–14 g/dl by the end of the procedure.

At the conclusion of the surgical procedure, the patient can usually be safely extubated, placed in a head up position, and transported on oxygen to the high dependency or intensive care unit.

POSTOPERATIVE CONSIDERATIONS

Careful assessment of the airway must be made during the early postoperative period. Most of the facial swelling, however, will be in the upper face and will not effect the airway. Postoperative blood loss can be substantial, but if adequate transfusion occurs intraoperatively, the haemoglobin on the first postoperative day should be about 10 g/dl. Analgesia is often satisfactory using non-opiate medication.

KEY POINTS

- There may be other congenital abnormalities associated with craniofacial abnormalities.
- Elevated ICP may be present.
- The airway may be difficult.
- Blood loss may be significant.
- Non-opioid analgesia is usually adequate postoperatively.

FURTHER READING

Ward CF. Pediatric head and neck syndromes. In: Katz J, Steward DJ (eds) Anesthesia and uncommon pediatric diseases, 2nd Edn. Philadelphia: WB Saunders, 1993, pp. 322–329

32

CONGENITAL SPINE LESIONS

J. Shapiro

INTRODUCTION

Congenital spinal defects result from the failure of the neural tube to close during the third or fourth week of gestation. The spectrum of defects ranges from spina bifida occulta, to myelomeningocoele, to anencephaly (failure of closure of the cephalad end of the neuro-tube). The most common lesions requiring surgical repair are the various forms of myelomeningocoele (MMC). The cause of MMC defects is multifactorial including both environmental (drug use, malnutrition, radiation) as well as a probable genetic predisposition. The incidence is thought to be about 1/1000 live births. However, in families with one affected child, the risk of recurrence is 3–4% and after two abnormal pregnancies, the risk approaches 10%. MMCs may occur anywhere along the neuroaxis, though the most common site is in the lumbosacral spine region.

CLINICAL FEATURES

Common manifestations include bowel and bladder dysfunction and varying degrees of motor and sensory loss below the spinal level of the lesion. Orthopaedic abnormalities are also common, including club foot and hip subluxation. Almost all patients with MMC develop hydrocephalus within the first month of life due to associated Arnold–Chiari malformations (displacement of the cerebellar vermis through the foramen magnum, elongation of the brainstem and fourth ventricle, and non-communicating hydrocephalus) and require CSF shunting procedures. Clinical examination usually reveals a midline cystic structure filled with CSF and neural elements. Often, the cyst is covered with a thin layer of epithelial cells and the terminus of the spinal cord (placoid). Despite the fact that this is a midline abnormality, there does not seem to be any relationship between MMCs and other congenital defects.

Two to three decades ago, attempts were made to determine which of these newborns should receive surgical treatment and which should be provided 'comfort care' in anticipation of imminent death. Several recent studies have confirmed that long-term survival of these patients is excellent, and their ability to function in society can be greatly enhanced with early repair and appropriate physiotherapy.

ANAESTHETIC MANAGEMENT

KEY PROBLEMS

1. *Risk of rupture of the cystic structure:* Loss of integrity of the MMC increases the risk of system infection or meningitis which may result in early mortality.
2. *Thermal loss:* In addition to the inability to adequately control their thermal environment, neonates are prone to evaporative thermal losses from the cyst.
3. *Airway management:* Patients are often intubated while in a lateral position to avoid pressure or traumatic injury to the defect. Postoperatively, the patient is supported in a prone or lateral position.

ASSESSMENT AND PREMEDICATION

Because neural tube defects do not appear to be associated with other congenital anomalies or syndromes, an in-depth assessment for cardiac, renal, or other systemic problems, which are not apparent at birth is probably not warranted. A thorough neurological assessment is, however, an essential component of the preoperative evaluation. It is important to remember that a prolonged delay in operative repair increases the risk of meningitis which carries a high mortality. Nevertheless, the usual assessment of cardiopulmonary systems and airway anatomy must be undertaken to assure that other issues do not result in perioperative complications. Prior to surgery, the neonate should be kept in a warm environment. Intravenous access should be obtained, and adequate i.v. hydration begun. In anticipation of surgery, the patient should remain nil by mouth. Positioning of the patient is of utmost importance. The neonate should be kept either prone or in a lateral position unless he can be supported in such a way as to avoid any contact or pressure on the cystic structure. Some sort of impervious dressing should be applied over the area of the defect to decrease the risk of infection. A bowel bag, similar to that used for omphalocoeles may be useful in this regard.

CONDUCT OF ANAESTHESIA

Following stabilisation after birth, the patient is brought to the operating theatre in a heated isolette to prevent hypothermia. Appropriate monitors including ECG, pulse oximetry, precordial stethoscope and non-invasive BP cuff are applied. Following induction, core temperature monitoring should also be added. If there are no obvious airway abnormalities, induction may proceed by either an inhalation technique with halothane or sevoflurane, or by i.v. agents such as thiopentone or propofol. Intubation is either accomplished with the patient in the lateral position, or, if supine, while being supported by foam pillows or towel rolls which ensure that the back is suspended above the operating table.

Short-acting muscle relaxants may be utilised to facilitate intubation if the practitioner prefers, but their use is not needed for the surgical procedure, and may interfere with the surgeon's ability to test for nerve root function during dissection and subsequent closure of the defect. Local anaesthetics are often used by the surgeon on the field. It is important to keep in mind acceptable doses so as to avoid overdose. Because the area of the lesion is usually relatively insensate, the use of narcotic analgesics is unnecessary and unwarranted unless closure requires a large musculocutaneous flap from above the lesion for coverage. Fluid requirements are the same as any other paediatric case, based on weight of the baby. Heat loss from the neonate should be minimised.

POSTOPERATIVE CONSIDERATIONS

As with all neonates (and particularly premature infants), the risk for apnoea and bradycardic spells following general anaesthesia exists. These patients should be monitored closely in an intensive care unit equipped and staffed to handle airway problems. Continued care to maintain a neutral thermal environment is essential. The patient is also observed for signs of irritability, nausea or vomiting, or decreased neurological function which might be indicative of hydrocephalus and increased ICP. Postoperative bleeding is seldom an issue if haemostasis is controlled at the time of closure. The patient is maintained in a horizontal position, either prone or lateral for several days until the dural closure has had an opportunity to begin healing. This decreases the risk of CSF leak or flap pressure ischaemia. If a CSF shunt is not placed at the time of initial surgery, these patients are usually returned to the operating theatre within the first postoperative week for placement of a V-P or ventriculo-atrial shunt to manage hydrocephalus.

KEY POINTS

- Early repair improves outcome in these children.
- Positioning is a common problem, and may complicate intubation.
- Narcotic analgesia is usually not required.
- Hydrocephalus may co-exist.
- Other major congenital abnormalities are not associated.
- Close postoperative observation is required for the first 2–3 days.

FURTHER READING

Krane EJ, Domino KB. Anesthesia for neurosurgery. In: Motoyama EK, Davis PJ (eds) Smith's anesthesia for infants and children. St Louis: CV Mosby, 1990

McLone DG. Congenital spinal cord anomalies. In: Menezes AH, Sonntag VKH (eds) Principles of spine surgery. New York: McGraw Hill, 1996

33

PAEDIATRIC CRANIOSPINAL TRAUMA

C. Duffy

PAEDIATRIC HEAD INJURIES

Head injuries account for over half of trauma-related deaths in children. The mechanism of injury is related to age, with infants suffering mainly falls and assaults while motor vehicle and bicycle accidents account for injuries in older children. Outcome after injury depends on:

- Admission GCS (or modified score for children; Chapter 36).
- Presence of epidural or subdural haematoma.
- Duration of coma.
- Multisystem trauma (with doubled mortality).

The paediatric brain responds differently to the adult brain when injured:

1. The relatively large head size and weak neck muscles render the child's brain more susceptible to acceleration–deceleration injuries.
2. Swelling is accommodated by skull expansion before the age of 2 and examination of the fontanelles and head circumference are important in the assessment of head injuries in this group. After this age, the skull sutures close and the cranial vault thickens.
3. Surgically treatable lesions are less common in children than in adults. Intracranial haematomas occur in 20–30% of paediatric head injuries, compared with 50% in adults. Due to the combination of a relatively small blood volume and large head size, scalp lacerations and intracranial haematomas may result in hypovolaemia and hypotension.
4. Children are less likely to have open skull fractures than adults because the calvarium is flexible and allow closed depressed skull fractures to occur.
5. Cerebral blood flow is thought to be higher in children than adults and tolerance to ischaemia *may* decrease as age increases. Overall, the functional outcome is better for children than for adults with a similar GCS on admission.

PATHOPHYSIOLOGY

Infants and children respond to head trauma initially with diffuse swelling lasting 1–2 days due to cerebral vasodilatation. Deterioration in a child after this time is more likely to be due to increased swelling or seizure activity than to a surgically treatable lesion. Post-traumatic seizures, even with minor head injuries, are more common in children aged < 2 years than in older patients. Prophylactic phenytoin (20 mg/kg) should be considered in a paralysed child when EEG monitoring is not available, especially in the younger child.

PREOPERATIVE MANAGEMENT

Neurological assessment is performed after adequate resuscitation. Persistent hypotension should alert to the possibility of associated injury (e.g. high cervical, abdominal or thoracic injury) or cervicomedullary injury with vasomotor centre damage.

Patients with a GCS ≤ 8 require urgent intubation with manual in-line stabilisation since up to 10% of paediatric head injuries are associated with cervical spine injuries. After intubation, the lungs are ventilated aiming for a $PaCO_2$ of 4–4.7 kPa, maintaining neutral head and neck position with head elevation of 15–20°. Diuretics are given with caution (e.g. mannitol 0.25–0.5 g/kg or furosemide 1 mg/kg) as diuresis can result in hypotension and electrolyte abnormalities. Mannitol can cause congestive heart failure in neonates. Therapeutic aims are for a CPP > 50 mmHg in infants and > 60 mmHg in older children. A CPP of < 40 mmHg is associated with a reduced survival rate (the normal ICP is 5 mmHg in infants and 10 mmHg in 5-year-olds). A CT scan can give an indication of prognosis. Subdural haematoma (evidence of severe trauma), ablated basal cisterns, midline shift and reversal of grey/white matter differentiation are all associated with a poor prognosis.

INTRAOPERATIVE MANAGEMENT

The aims of intraoperative management have been outlined in Chapter 12, i.e. maintaining adequate anaesthesia, analgesia, sedation, muscle paralysis and cerebral perfusion together with ventilation to a $PaCO_2$ of 4–4.7 kPa, mild hypothermia (34–36°C), normovolaemia, an appropriate haematocrit for the patient's age and underlying medical condition and a normal blood sugar. An ICP monitor can be inserted intraoperatively and used as a guide to ensure CPP is adequate. Destruction of brain tissue can cause release of thromboplastin and lead to DIC. Coagulopathy should be treated with appropriate haemostatic factors.

POSTOPERATIVE MANAGEMENT

Due to the risk of early cerebral vasodilatation, patients who have required surgical intervention are ventilated with ICP monitoring in the immediate postoperative period. Further neuroprotective strategies are considered in severe head injury (Chapter 40).

PAEDIATRIC SPINAL INJURIES

Spinal injuries are usually due to motor vehicle accidents in younger children, either as a pedestrian or passenger. In older children, they tend to result from falls or diving accidents. More than one spinal level is affected in up to 20% of paediatric spinal injuries.

Like the paediatric brain, the paediatric spine responds differently to the adult spine when injured. Ligamentous laxity and incomplete bony ossification protect the child against spinal injury but increase the likelihood of subluxation without fractures and SCIWORA (spinal cord injury without obvious radiological abnormality). SCIWORA occurs in 20–60% of spinal injuries. Clinical suspicion or equivocal radiology should be treated as spinal injury until definitive tests (e.g. CT, MRI) have been performed.

Neck movement has greater momentum than in adults due to the relatively large head and poor neck muscle support. The fulcrum of mobility is at C2–3 in children and C4–5 in adults. Injuries between the occiput and C2 account for 40% of paediatric spinal injuries, compared with 20% in adults.

PATHOPHYSIOLOGY

Spinal cord injury can be suspected in the unconscious patient with unexplained hypotension and bradycardia, priapism, flaccidity, immobility and arreflexia below level of lesion, apnoea for lesions at or above C3, impaired ventilation for lesions at or above C5 and paradoxical respiration from paralysed intercostal muscles for lesions below C6. Spinal shock occurs for the first 3–5 days following injury followed by autonomic hyperreflexia. Other systemic effects include paralytic ileus, urinary retention and poikilothermia below the level of the lesion.

PREOPERATIVE MANAGEMENT

Urgent neurosurgical intervention is required to reduce and stabilise the spine where conservative measures are unlikely to succeed; to decompress ± fuse the spine in a neurologically deteriorating patient; and for non-spinal surgery for associated injuries. Early administration of methylprednisolone has been shown to improve clinical outcome at 6 weeks and 6 months post-injury. A dose of 30 mg/kg should be given within 8 hours of injury followed by 5.4 mg/kg/h for the next 23 hours.

INTRAOPERATIVE MANAGEMENT

Manual in-line stabilisation performed with an assistant applying gentle traction to the mastoid processes should be used to secure the airway. Padding under the torso keeps the head position neutral. Splinting the head and torso to a board with sandbags on either side of the neck helps reduce mobility. Adequate sedation and muscle relaxant are given to aid intubation. Suxamethonium can be given safely within 48 hours of spinal injury. After 48 hours, the risk of hyperkalaemia precludes the use of suxamethonium. Once the airway is secured, aim for adequate anaesthesia, analgesia, sedation, muscle paralysis and cord perfusion together with ventilation to a $PaCO_2$ of 4–4.7 kPa, normovolaemia, mild hypothermia, a normal haematocrit and a normal blood sugar.

Both the surgeon and anaesthetist should position the patient. Neutral head and neck position should be maintained during transfer to the operating table. Patients are positioned so that there is free diaphragmatic excursion and minimal venous congestion at the surgical site. Bony prominences, eyes and nose should be protected. Traction on peripheral nerves should be minimised. Blood pressure should be maintained at preoperative levels using CVP and urine output as a guide to volume status. Any bradycardia should be treated with anticholinergic agents.

POSTOPERATIVE MANAGEMENT

Ventilation should be continued postoperatively when respiration has been impaired preoperatively. In the early postoperative period, sedation can be lightened in order to assess adequacy of cough, ventilation and neurological function.

KEY POINTS

- Mechanisms of head and spinal injuries in children differ from adult injury.
- Target CPP is lower in infants compared to older children and adults.
- Adequate fluid resuscitation is of paramount importance.
- Cervical spine injuries are more likely to be at a higher level in children.

FURTHER READING

Simpson D, Reilly P. Paediatric coma scale (letter). Lancet 1982; 2: 450

Muizelaar JP, Marmarou AM, DeSalles AA, et al. Cerebral blood flow in severely head injured children. Part 1: Relationship with GCS score, outcome, ICP and PVI. J Neurosurg 1989; 71: 63–71

Muizelaar JP, Ward JD, Marmarou AM, et al. Cerebral blood flow in severely head injured children. Part II: Autoregulation. J Neurosurg 1989; 71: 72–76

Bracken MB, Shepherd MJ, Collins WF, et al. A random-ized, controlled trial of methylprednisolone or naloxone in the treatment of acute spinal-cord injury. N Engl J Med 1990: 322: 1405–1411

American Heart Association. Pediatric Advanced Life Support. Trauma Resus 1997: 8–3

Ward JD. Pediatric issues in head trauma. New Horizons 1995; 3: 539–545

34

RECOVERY: GENERAL CONSIDERATIONS

S. Gupta

INTRODUCTION

There is perhaps no other branch of surgery where a postoperative complication has such a devastating effect. The post-anaesthesia care of the neurosurgical patient requires careful monitoring, exquisite attention to maintenance of cardiorespiratory stability and frequent neurological assessment. Appropriate staff, equipment and monitoring is mandatory for proper care of patients.

AIRWAY AND VENTILATION

Hypoxia or hypercapnia may result from hypoventilation due to residual neuromuscular blockade, perioperative use of opioids, electrolyte imbalance or brainstem compression due to oedema or haematoma. Hypoventilation will increase ICP and impair brain oxygenation.

Patients with good GCS scores who are haemodynamically stable with adequate oxygenation preoperatively may be extubated following neurosurgery if the intraoperative course has been uneventful. Normothermia and adequate neuromuscular reversal are prerequisites to extubation.

Protective airway reflexes may be compromised for a variety of reasons, in particular cranial nerve injury or depressed level of consciousness.

The airway may be compressed by haematoma after cervical spine or carotid surgery causing stridor and hypoxia.

CENTRAL NERVOUS SYSTEM

Postoperatively, altered level of consciousness could be either due to residual effects of anaesthetic drugs or more commonly cerebral pathology. Close observation of GCS is necessary to detect any changes that may occur in the postoperative period. Focal signs such as change in pupillary size are a good indicator of an evolving postoperative complication, e.g. intracranial haematoma. Haemodynamic changes such as hypertension and bradycardia (Cushing's response) or altered ventilatory pattern are also important signs of possible postoperative complications. If a complication is suspected then immediate CT scanning is indicated to rapidly diagnose a reversible problem which may be resolved surgically.

If seizures occur postoperatively control should be obtained with small doses of benzodiazipines while ensuring an adequate airway. A CT scan should be performed to determine any focal lesion and if a patient's GCS does not improve after the post-ictal period an EEG should be performed and anticonvulsants commenced.

CARDIOVASCULAR SYSTEM

Uncontrolled hypertension during emergence and recovery has been implicated as a causative factor of postoperative intracranial haemorrhage after aneurysm clipping.[1] Patients with atherosclerosis are likely to be hypertensive preoperatively, and may be more susceptible to postoperative hypertension.

If there is no apparent primary cause of hypertension, aggressive efforts at control are warranted because of the risk that hypertension will precipitate haemorrhage or worsen cerebral oedema. Treatment consists of administering titrated doses of either labetalol (5–10 mg increments i.v.), small doses of esmolol or sublingual nifedipine (10–20 mg).

Patients with cerebrovascular or cardiovascular disease are also susceptible to large variations in BP, both hypertension and hypotension. This will increase the likelihood of cerebral or myocardial ischaemia or infarction.

NAUSEA AND VOMITING

Postoperative nausea and vomiting may increase BP and ICP. Droperidol, 0.625–2.5 mg intravenously, promethazine 12.5–25 mg i.v. or intramuscularly Cyclizine 50 mg i.v. or Ondansatron 4–8 mg i.v. may be used to control nausea and vomiting. Refractory nausea may suggest development of acute hydrocephalus or increased ICP secondary to brain oedema or haematoma.

FLUID AND ELECTROLYTE BALANCE

Fluid loss and intake are carefully noted with the aim of maintaining normovolaemia except in patient's following aneurysm clipping in whom hypervolaemic haemodilution is preferred.

Electrolytes should be measured early in the postoperative period to monitor changes in serum sodium and potassium, particularly if diuretics have been administered. If a suprasellar mass has been resected or the patient has experienced severe head injury, the onset of diabetes insipidus should be considered if urinary output exceeds 200–400 ml/h and if specific gravity is less than 1.005 and be treated by administering vasopressin or DDAVP (1 μg). The syndrome of inappropriate secretion of ADH is associated with CNS trauma or tumour. Diagnosis and treatment of electrolyte and fluid balance abnormalities are described in Chapters 42 and 43.

POSTOPERATIVE PAIN

Postoperative pain is controlled by regular doses of paracetamol and NSAID (if no contraindications exist) supplemented either by carefully titrated doses of codeine phosphate or morphine sulphate ensuring against excessive sedation. Nausea and vomiting due to opioids should be treated promptly.

DISCHARGE

Patients should not be discharged to the surgical wards until an adequate conscious level has returned fully, a patent airway can be maintained, ventilation is adequate and the cardiovascular system is stable.

Patients whose GCS is compromised and/or whose ability to maintain an airway is in doubt should not be extubated immediately postoperatively and should be transferred to an intensive care environment. Patients who have had intracranial vascular surgery, prolonged posterior fossa surgery or carotid artery surgery should be nursed in a high dependency area with invasive monitoring for at least 24 hours.

PERSONNEL AND MONITORING

Recovery personnel experienced in assessing the CNS are central to an adequate recovery facility. Invasive arterial monitoring and pulse oximetry should be continuous from the operating room to the recovery room and during the patient's stay in recovery. Full monitoring should also continue when transferred to ICU. An experienced anaesthetist should also be immediately available while a patient remains in the recovery area.

KEY POINTS

- Recovery personnel should be experienced in neurological assessment.
- Any deterioration in neurology should be rapidly assessed and investigated.
- Correction of fluid and electrolyte balance can continue in recovery.
- Adequate analgesia should be established prior to discharge.
- A detailed handover between recovery and ward staff is essential.

REFERENCE

1. Kalfas IH, Little JR. Postoperative haemorrhage: a survey of 4992 intracranial procedures. Neurosurgery 1988; 23: 343

Section 5

NEUROINTENSIVE CARE

35

MANAGEMENT OF SPINAL CORD INJURY

I. Ng, R. J. C. Laing

INTRODUCTION

The management of patients with spinal cord injury requires a multi-disciplinary approach to achieve maximal neurological recovery and to prevent, recognise and treat any complications.

Mortality is at its highest in the early stages of treatment and most patients with spinal cord injury have other associated injuries.

An understanding of the pathophysiological processes has led to a more rational approach to spinal cord injury, with the main thrust aimed at prevention of cord ischaemia and worsening secondary injury and more recently, the use of steroids to reduce the harmful effects of lipid peroxidation.

PATHOPHYSIOLOGY

The *primary injury* is the immediate damage inflicted on the spinal cord and is due to either impact with compression (e.g. disc rupture, burst fracture or fracture dislocation), impact without compression (hyperextension injuries), distraction (burst fracture) or cord laceration. Any loss of neuronal tissue is likely to be permanent.

The *secondary injury* comprises all damage that occurs to the cord following the initial impact and is potentially preventable by prompt resuscitation and good intensive care.

Systemic Effects of Spinal Cord Injury

Neurogenic or spinal shock (see below) results in the secondary loss of sympathetic tone, and together with unopposed vagotonia leads to a state of systemic hypotension that is related to the level and severity of injury. This state of hypoperfusion leads to cord ischaemia which will compound the injury already sustained.

Local Effects

Vascular changes

Damage to the microvasculature including both capillaries and venules, results in microhaemorrhages and thrombosis. The spinal cord at the level of the injury undergoes infarction as the neurones at the epicentre of the injury become ischaemic.

Biochemical changes

With the disruption of the integrity of the neural tissue, the Na^+/K^+ pump fails with accumulation of intracellular sodium and resultant cytotoxic oedema.

The release of glutamate activates NMDA receptors resulting in an influx of calcium. This causes activation of calcium-dependent proteases and lipases that break down the cytoskeleton. The excess production of arachidonic acid and its metabolites and consequent lipid peroxidation and free radical production leads to further injury.

Current research into the mechanisms of injury has led to the use of methylprednisolone to lessen the effects of lipid peroxidation (see below). Further research is being conducted to establish the effectiveness of other agents in modifying the pathophysiological processes which contribute to spinal cord injury at the molecular level. The aims are to promote neuronal salvage and ultimately improve clinical outcome.

DIAGNOSIS

The diagnosis of spinal cord injury requires a high index of suspicion on the part of the attending physician. These patients often have other more life-threatening conditions that divert attention away from the spinal cord injury. All patients with head injury are assumed to have a cervical injury until proven otherwise. A cervical collar should be fitted until definitive investigation has taken place. The mechanism of injury may give a clue to the likely presence of a spinal injury, for example the association between rear seat lap strap restraint and thoraco-lumbar burst fractures.

Careful neurological examination should include an assessment of tone, reflexes, motor power and sensation if possible. The anal tone should be checked and patients should be log-rolled to allow examination of the back. The presence of bruising or a palpable step in the spine may indicate an underlying spinal injury. In the conscious trauma patient, the complaint of pain in any part of the spine must be taken seriously and if plain X-rays are normal further radiological assessment is necessary. Spinal shock refers to the complete loss of motor, tone, sensory and reflex activity below the affected spinal segment. It may last as long as 6 weeks. The end of spinal shock is heralded by the return of spinal reflexes.

Computed axial tomography is very sensitive to the presence of bony injury but further investigation with MRI may be required to diagnose ligamentous injury and soft tissue encroachment into the spinal canal. Flexion and extension cervical spine films will diagnose the presence of ligamentous instability. Although usually safe in the conscious patient they should only be ordered by experienced doctors following full assessment of the mechanism of injury and the static radiological images.

ASSOCIATED INJURIES AND MANAGEMENT ISSUES

Sixty per cent of patients with spinal cord injuries have associated injuries: head, thoracic, abdominal or vascular injuries. This underlies the importance of meticulous initial assessment and subsequent regular review of the patient.

CARDIOVASCULAR

The presence of hypotension may indicate neurogenic shock with loss of sympathetic innervation to the heart and peripheral vasculature. Hypovolaemic hypotension secondary to concealed or overt blood loss may be concurrent and useful indicators are unexplained tachycardia with narrowed pulse pressure. Aggressive fluid resuscitation is necessary to prevent further injury. Invasive haemodynamic monitoring may be indicated to guide fluid and inotrope therapy.

PULMONARY FUNCTION

Respiratory dysfunction following spinal cord injuries occurs from loss of neural control of ventilatory muscles (high cervical injuries) or is secondary to parenchymal injury, e.g. pulmonary contusion, pneumothorax, haemothorax, atelectasis, neurogenic pulmonary oedema, adult respiratory distress syndrome, fat embolism, pulmonary embolism or aspiration.

Patients requiring mechanical ventilation need active chest physiotherapy including suction, humidification and bronchodilators to prevent retention of secretions and optimise gas exchange.

Early tracheostomy for patients with multiple injuries and pulmonary dysfunction is strongly advocated.

NUTRITION

Patients with spinal cord injury are often in a catabolic state and therefore feeding should be started as soon as possible. Enteral feeding via an indwelling nasogastric tube is the method of choice. Patients with associated abdominal injuries or those with ileus secondary to cord injury (thoraco-lumbar injuries), may require parenteral nutrition.

BLADDER

During the acute period of spinal cord injury, the bladder is atonic. An indwelling urinary catheter will prevent bladder distension and allows accurate monitoring of fluid output.

DECUBITUS ULCERS

Direct pressure on weight-bearing areas, sensory loss, reduced mobility and reduced tissue perfusion expose the patient to a high risk of skin breakdown. This can be prevented by careful nursing with frequent turning of patients. Padding of pressure areas with soft foam or nursing on oscillating or air flotation beds can help prevent this problem.

SURGICAL TREATMENT

Intuitively, it would be expected that the surgical decompression of bony fragments encroaching on neural elements would result in improved neurological outcome. Many reports have been published that show that emergency attempts at surgical decompression have led to a worse outcome than patients treated conservatively. This may be due to problems of inadequate resuscitation pre and per-operatively and complications secondary to poorly planned or executed surgery. Operative treatment can restore normal spinal alignment, allow early mobilisation and prevent delayed deformity. Emergency decompression may be indicated for cord compression without laceration due to disc fragments in the canal. Most spinal surgeons therefore adopt a more conservative approach with delayed surgical decompression and spinal stabilisation when indicated. The stabilisation procedure with bone grafting and instrumentation facilitates nursing.

METHYLPREDNISOLONE THERAPY

The results of the NASCIS III trial[1] have shown that patients arriving within 3 hours and given a bolus dose of 30 mg/kg methylprednisolone followed by 5.4 mg/kg/h for 24 hours, as well as patients who arrive between 3 and 8 hours after injury and having had the same loading dose followed by 48 hours of methylprenisolone, have improved motor scores and better functional independence scores at 1 year post-injury compared to patients receiving no methylprednisolone. Patients who arrive later than 8 hours do not derive any benefit from methylprednisolone treatment.

KEY POINTS

• Spinal cord injury should be suspected after major trauma.

- The management of spinal cord injury requires early aggressive resuscitation to prevent systemic hypotension.
- The use of methylprednisolone in patients who arrive within the 8-hour therapeutic window should be considered.
- Delayed surgical decompression and stabilisation should be considered in suitable candidates.

FURTHER READING

Geisler WO, Jousee AT, Wynne-Jones M. Survival in traumatic transverse myelitis. Paraplegia 1977; 14: 262

Tator CH. Pathophysiology and pathology of spinal cord injury. In: Wilkins RH, Rengachary SS (eds) Neurosurgery, Vol 2. New York: McGraw Hill, 1996, pp. 2847–2859

Frisbie JH, Sarkarati M, Sharma GV, Rossier AB. Venous thrombosis and pulmonary embolism occurring at close intervals in spinal cord injury patients. Paraplegia 1983; 21: 270–271

Grahm TW, Zadrozny DB, Harrington T. The benefits of early jejunal hyperalimentation in the head-injured patient. Neurosurgery 1989; 25: 729–735

Marshall LF, Knowlton S, Garfin SR, et al. Deterioration following spinal cord injury. A multicenter study. J Neurosurg 1987; 66: 400–404

REFERENCE

1. Bracken MB, Shepard MJ, Holford TR, et al. Methylprednisolone or tirilazad mesylate administration after acute spinal cord injury: 1-year follow up. Results of the third National Acute Spinal Cord Injury randomized controlled trial. J Neurosurg 1998; 89: 699–706

36

GLASGOW COMA SCALE

A. Summors

INTRODUCTION

The Glasgow coma scale (GCS) in adults (Table 36.1) is a method of continuous rapid neurological assessment and is commonly used in the acutely brain-injured patient and perioperatively in neurosurgical patients. It may also help as a prognostic indicator.

Scores range from 3 to 15. Scores less than 9 usually indicate a requirement for airway and ventilatory support and ICP monitoring.

In children, a modified GCS can be obtained using the same scores for eye opening and best motor response and a modified best verbal response (Table 36.2).

A Glasgow coma outcome scale (GCOS) (Table 36.3) of function is commonly performed 6 months following traumatic brain injury. This allows individual centres to compare results and to compare new therapies.

FURTHER READING

Teasdale C, Jennet B. Assessment and prognosis of coma after head injury. Acta Neurochir (Wien) 1976; 34: 45–55

Table 36.1 Glasgow coma scale

Eye opening:	Spontaneous	4
	To speech	3
	To pain	2
	None	1
Best motor response:	Obeys commands	6
	Localises to pain	5
	Withdraws to pain	4
	Abnormal flexion	3
	Extension	2
	None	1
Best verbal response:	Orientated	5
	Confused	4
	Inappropriate words	3
	Incomprehensible sounds	2
	None	1

Table 36.3 Glasgow Coma Outcome Scale

Good recovery	4
Moderately disabled (disabled but independent)	3
Severely disabled (disabled and dependent)	2
Died	1

Table 36.2 Modified paediatric GCS

Eye opening:	Spontaneous		4
	To speech		3
	To pain		2
	None		1
Best motor response:	Obeys commands		6
	Localises to pain		5
	Withdraws to pain		4
	Abnormal flexion		3
	Extension		2
	None		1
Best verbal response	Smiles, follows objects, interacts		5
	Crying:	*Interaction:*	
	Consolable	Inappropriate	4
	Inconsistently Consolable	Moaning	3
	Inconsolable	Irritable	2
	None	None	1

37

SEVERE HEAD INJURY: INITIAL RESUSCITATION AND TRANSFER

B. Matta

INTRODUCTION

Although better pre-hospital care and the ready availability of multi-disciplinary teams have improved the very poor outlook that was previously associated with head trauma, outcome continues to be affected by abnormal physiology in the immediate post-injury period.

The *primary injury*, which is not treatable and can only be prevented, describes the damage that occurs at the time of initial impact. Severe HI renders the patient comatose from impact; those able to talk at any stage following the injury are unlikely to have sustained a substantial primary injury.

Secondary injury is the additional insult imposed on the neural tissue following the primary impact. The two most important contributors to secondary ischaemia in the head-injured patient are hypoxaemia and systemic hypotension.

INITIAL RESUSCITATION

The importance of securing the airway, maintaining adequate oxygenation and BP in the head-injured patient cannot be over-emphasised. Secondary brain damage begins and continues to occur from the moment of impact and for every second that the patient is hypoxaemic or hypotensive. Severely head-injured patients (GCS < 9) are unlikely to be able to protect their airway and often have impaired gas exchange. Early use of endotracheal intubation is often necessary to maintain adequate oxygenation. It is important to remember that a significant proportion of severe HIs are associated with injuries to the cervical spine and therefore, manual in-line stabilisation of the neck during induction and tracheal intubation is *essential*. Nasal intubation is best avoided in the patient with basal skull fracture because of the risk of passing the endotracheal tube into the brain through the skull defect, and of the added risk of infection.

Severely head-injured patients have a full stomach. Therefore, a rapid sequence induction with a small dose of induction agent followed by suxamethonium 1 mg/kg is mandatory. Apart from ketamine, which is contraindicated because of concerns about its effects on ICP, the choice of induction agent is not important as long as it is administered with care and large variations in BP or significant hypotension is avoided.

Once the airway is secured, the lungs are mechanically ventilated to maintain mild hypocapnia (not less than 4 kPa) and an adequate PaO_2. Oxygenation and ventilation is optimised and should be regularly verified by arterial blood gas analysis. The patient is best sedated and paralysed. Patients should not cough or strain on the endotracheal tube. Clearly, not all patients with head trauma require tracheal intubation, and the protocol used in our unit is outlined in Table 37.1.

Except for young children, in whom blood loss from a scalp wound is sufficient to cause a reduced MAP, hypotension should prompt an investigation for sites of blood loss with immediate laparotomy or thoracotomy if necessary. The combination of an increased ICP and systemic hypotension leads to cerebral ischaemia. Hypovolaemia may be masked by systemic hypertension secondary to intense sympathetic stimulation of the reflex response to intracranial hypertension. Therefore, moderate levels of hypertension should not be treated but a BP above the upper limit of autoregulation (MAP > 130 mmHg) must be actively treated, as it will increase CBV and ICP.

The choice of fluid used for resuscitation is less important than the amount given. The use of glucose-containing solutions is discouraged unless hypoglycaemia is suspected, as hyperglycaemia worsens

---

Table 37.1 Indications for intubation and ventilation after head injury

Immediately
- Coma (not obeying commands, not speaking, not eye opening i.e. GCS < 9)
- Loss of protective laryngeal reflexes
- Ventilatory insufficiency as judged by blood gases:
    Hypoxaemia (PaO_2 < 13 kPa)
    Spontaneous hyperventilation causing $PaCO_2$ < 3.5 kPa
- Respiratory arrhythmia
- Uncontrolled seizures

Before start of journey to the neurointensive care unit
- Deteriorating level of consciousness (decrease in GCS by > 2 points since admission, and not due to drugs), even if not in coma
- Bilaterally fractured mandible
- Copious bleeding into mouth (e.g. from a basal skull fracture)
- Seizures

An intubated patient must also be ventilated, aiming for a PaO_2 > 13 kPa and $PaCO_2$ of 4.0–4.5 kPa.

outcome after HI. Hyperglycaemia should be actively treated and blood glucose levels controlled with an infusion of insulin. Because the majority of head-injured patients receive mannitol, an adequate urine output is often a poor indicator of volume status in these patients. CVP monitoring is often very useful as an aid to assessing intravascular fluid volume and effectiveness of resuscitation, and should be combined with the use of a pulmonary artery flotation catheter in the elderly, patients with heart disease and in those patients requiring the use of inotropic support.

TRANSFER OF THE HEAD-INJURED PATIENT

Adequate resuscitation and a thorough re-examination of the patient must be completed before making decisions about further treatment priorities. Blind burrhole exploration is rarely effective, can be harmful to the patient, and delays the transfer of the patient and the initiation of definitive therapy. There is no longer any indication for this procedure in the modern Accident and Emergency Department. Once the patient has been stabilised, a decision can be made regarding transfer to a regional neurosurgical unit for further treatment. Inter-hospital transfer of the head-injured patient is a potentially hazardous procedure and often poorly managed (Table 37.2). The key to a successful and safe transfer involves:

- Adequate resuscitation and stabilisation of the patient prior to transfer.
- Adequate monitoring during transfer with appropriate resuscitative equipment and drugs.
- The presence of an accompanying doctor with suitable training, skills and experience of HI transfer.
- Good communication between referring and receiving centres, and an adequate, efficient and stable hand-over to the receiving team care.

The fundamental requirement during transfer is to ensure adequate tissue oxygen delivery and to maintain stable perfusion. The head-injured patient is at risk of respiratory compromise, and this risk is increased during transfer. Patients with a significantly altered conscious level should be sedated, intubated and ventilated during transfer. *There is no place for transferring unstable patients to neurosurgical units.*

The transferring team must ensure that all lines and tubes are secured before transfer, that they have a

Table 37.2 What the neurosurgical centre needs to know at time of referral

Patient's age and past medical history (if known)
History of injury
- Time of Injury
- Cause and mechanism (height of fall, approximate impact velocity)
Neurological state
- Talked or not after injury
- Consciousness level on arrival at A&E dept
- Trends in consciousness level after arrival (sequential GCS)
- Pupil and limb responses
Cardiorespiratory state
- Blood pressure and pulse rate
- Arterial blood gases, respiratory rate and pattern
Injuries
- Skull fracture
- Extracranial injuries
Imaging findings
- Haematoma, swelling, other
Management
- Airway protection, ventilatory status
- Circulatory status and fluid therapy (Mannitol)
- Treatment of associated injuries (? emergency surgery)
- Monitoring
- Drug doses and times of administration

sufficient supply of drugs and portable gases, and that there is enough power in battery-operated monitoring equipment for the duration of the journey.

Monitoring during transfer should be of a standard appropriate to a patient in intensive care, and should include invasive arterial BP monitoring, CVP monitoring where indicated, and the use of capnography. The transferring doctor must have appropriate experience in the transfer of patients with HIs, should be familiar with the pathophysiology and management of such a patient, and with the drugs and equipment they will use. It is also of paramount importance to discuss the patient with the neurosurgical centre at an early stage, so that treatment priorities can be decided upon, and that the receiving team is prepared for the arrival of the patient. The care of the transferring doctor does not end at the door of the receiving hospital, but continues until he ensures that the stability of the patient is maintained and a full and accurate hand-over to the receiving team is made.

KEY POINTS

- Hypotension and hypoxia are two major contributors to secondary brain injury and should be avoided.
- The cervical spine should be assumed to be unstable until cleared by radiological examination.
- Rapid resuscitation and adequate stabilisation is essential prior to transfer.
- Good communication between the referring centre and the neurosurgical centre is required.
- Appropriate personnel, equipment and monitoring should accompany the patient.

FURTHER READING

Matta BF, Menon DK. Management of acute head injury: pathophysiology and initial resuscitation. Anaes Rev 1995; 13: 163–178

Matta BF, Menon DK. Severe head injury in the United Kingdom and Ireland: a survey of practice and implications for management. Crit Care Med 1996; 24: 1743–1748

Gentleman D, Dearden M, Midgley S, Maclean D. Guidelines for the resuscitation and transfer of patients with serious head injury. Br Med J 1993; 307: 547–552

The Association of Anaesthetists of Great Britain and Ireland. Recommendations on transfer of the severely head injured patient

38

INTENSIVE CARE MANAGEMENT OF ACUTE HEAD INJURY

D.K. Menon

DETERMINANTS OF OUTCOME IN ACUTE HEAD INJURY:
PRIMARY VS SECONDARY INSULTS

Little can be done about the extent of primary injury following head trauma, but secondary neuronal injury, much of which is triggered by physiological insults to the injured brain, can be a major determinant of outcome. The most important physiological insults that affect outcome (Table 38.1) can be graded for severity with respect to their effect on secondary neuronal injury. Physiological insults are additive in their effect on outcome, both when multiple insults (e.g. hypoxia and hypotension) occur at the same time point, or when the same insult occurs repeatedly (e.g. hypotension in the prehospital and ICU phases of the illness). The intensive care of head injury centres on avoiding, detecting and treating such physiological derangements.

Targets for basic intensive care practice in this area have been widely debated and systematically reviewed. These involve the monitoring, prevention and treatment of secondary physiological insults. Novel neuroprotective agents may hold considerable promise in the future, but their general failure in clinical phase III suggests that these drugs are unlikely to materially alter outcome in the short term.

However, there appears to be much room for improvement in conventional clinical practice. A series of surveys suggest that basic recommendations for severe head injury management have not been consistently followed in many neurosurgical centres in the USA and UK. As an example, ICP was monitored in only half the centres surveyed. While preliminary results suggest that this situation may now be improving, the application of novel neuroprotective therapies is futile if stable cardiorespiratory and cerebrovascular physiology cannot be achieved.

MONITORING IN ACUTE HEAD INJURY

None of the interventions that are widely used by specialist centres in severe head injury have ever been subjected to prospective randomised control trials, but a large body of clinical experience provides a relatively strong basis for their recommendation as treatment guidelines.

DEFINING THERAPEUTIC TARGETS: A RATIONAL APPROACH TO SELECTING MONITORING MODALITIES

Basic physiology suggests the benefit of maintaining CBF and oxygenation. Hypotension (systolic blood pressure < 90 mmHg) and hypoxia (PaO_2 levels < 60 mmHg (8 kPa)) in the early and later phases of head injury worsen outcome. Several studies in patients with head injury have suggested preserved cerebrovascular autoregulation with maintenance of CBF at CPP above 60–70 mmHg. Further, ischaemia is a consistent post-mortem finding in fatal head injury, and retrospective studies from several groups have suggested that outcome is improved in patients who have fewer episodes of CPP or MAP reduction or aggressive CPP management. There is, however, some emerging concern that relatively high perfusion pressures may contribute to oedema formation, and at least one group have targeted relatively low CPP in order to minimise oedema formation (the Lund protocol). Other small studies show worse outcomes in patients who suffer episodes of jugular venous

Table 38.1 Physiological insults following head injury and their relation to outcome		
Insult	Significant relation to	
	Mortality	Grades within Glasgow outcome score
Duration of hypotension (SBP $\leq$ 90 mmHg)	Yes	Yes
Duration of hypoxia (SpO$_2$ $\leq$ 90%)	Yes	No
Duration of pyrexia (T$_{core}$ $\geq$ 38°C)	Yes	No
Intracranial hypertension (ICP > 30 mmHg)	Yes	No
Cerebral perfusion pressure (CPP < 50 mmHg)	Yes	No

desaturation below 50%, or blood glucose elevation. Elevations in body temperature may worsen outcome in acute brain injury.

These findings emphasise the importance of maintenance of CPP, rather than isolated attention to ICP as a therapeutic target. There are, however, data that show that ICP is an independent, albeit weaker, determinant of outcome in severe head injury, with levels greater than 15–25 mmHg constituting an appropriate threshold for initiation of therapy.

MONITORING SYSTEMIC PHYSIOLOGY

Monitoring of direct arterial blood pressure along with measurement of ICP is essential for computing and manipulating CPP. The need to rationally manipulate mean arterial pressure will also require the placement of a right atrial or pulmonary artery catheter as appropriate. Continuous pulse oximetry, regular arterial blood gas analysis, core temperature monitoring and regular measurement of blood sugar are also required in order to optimise physiology in these patients.

GLOBAL CNS MONITORING MODALITIES

While the monitoring described above may help to ensure the maintenance of optimal systemic physiology, detection of local changes in CNS physiology will require other tools. These include transcranial Doppler ultrasound for non-invasive estimation of CBF, jugular venous saturation (SjvO$_2$) monitoring, and monitoring of brain electrical activity. These techniques seek to estimate CBF in the presence of an adequate CPP, estimate the adequacy of oxygen delivery to the brain, and document the consequences of possible oxygen deficit or drug therapy on brain function respectively.

ICP MONITORING

ICP monitoring is needed because clinical signs of intracranial hypertension are late, inconsistent and non-specific. Further, it has been shown that episodic rises in ICP may occur even in patients with a normal X-ray CT scan. While intraparenchymal micromanometers (Codman, USA) or fibreoptic probes (Camino, USA) are increasingly used due to ease of use and a lower infection risk, they are more expensive than ventriculostomies and do not permit CSF drainage for the reduction of elevated ICP.

Patients with head injury may also develop phasic increases in ICP, often triggered by cerebral vasodilatation in response to a fall in CPP. 'A waves' tend to occur on a high baseline pressure and elevate ICP to 50–100 mmHg for several minutes, usually terminated by a marked increase in mean arterial pressure. Shorter lived fluctuations lasting about a minute are referred to as B waves. The frequency of both A and B waves may be decreased by increasing MAP, thus preventing the reflex cerebral vasodilatory cascade that initiates CBV increases and ICP elevation (see Chapter 52 for further information).

TCD ULTRASONOGRAPHY

Reductions in middle cerebral artery flow velocity (MCA FV) provide a useful marker of reduced cerebral perfusion in the setting of intracranial hypertension, but episodic rises in ICP may also be caused by hyperaemia, which may be diagnosed by *increases* in TCD FV. Transcranial Doppler ultrasonography can also be used as a non-invasive monitor of CPP.

Tests of autoregulation involve recording TCD responses to induced changes in mean arterial pressure or carotid compression (the transient hyperaemic response test; THRT). More recent algorithms constantly assess autoregulation by on-line calculation of changes in MCA FV in response to small spontaneous alterations in MAP.

JUGULAR VENOUS OXIMETRY

Classically, right jugular venous oximetry has been used to assess the adequacy of CBF in head injury, but a case can be made for targeting the side of injury or for using bilateral catheterisation. Reductions in SjvO$_2$ or increases in arteriojugular differences in oxygen content (AJDO$_2$) to greater than 9 ml/dl provide useful markers of inadequate CBF, and SjvO$_2$ values below 50% have been shown to be associated with a worse outcome in head injury. Conversely, marked elevations in SjvO$_2$ may provide evidence of cerebral hyperaemia. The major deficiencies of jugular venous oximetry are its invasiveness and the poor reliability of signal obtained. Other techniques that have been employed investigationally in acute head injury include near infra-red spectroscopy (NIRS), direct tissue oximetry and cerebral microdialysis.

MULTIMODALITY MONITORING

The correlation of data from several modalities has several advantages in head injury management. Integration of monitored variables allows cross validation and artifact rejection, better understanding of pathophysiology and the potential to target therapy.

THERAPY

ACHIEVING TARGET CPP VALUES

Most centres agree on the need to maintain cerebral perfusion by keeping CPP above 60–70 mmHg, either by decreasing ICP or by increasing MAP. While MAP is usually maintained with volume expansion, inotropes and vasopressors, the relative efficiency of each of these interventions in maintaining CPP have not been investigated. Drainage of CSF (where possible), mannitol administration, hyperventilation and the use of CNS depressants (typically barbiturates) have all been used to reduce ICP.

VENTILATORY SUPPORT AND THE USE OF HYPOCAPNIA FOR ICP REDUCTION

It is generally agreed that patients with a GCS of ≤ 8 require intubation for airway protection, and that such patients should receive mechanical ventilatory support to optimise blood gases. Airway control and ventilation are also required for patients with ventilatory failure, central neurogenic hyperventilation or recurrent fits.

Hyperventilation, once the mainstay of ICP reduction in severe head injury, is now the subject of much debate. The aim of hyperventilation is to reduce cerebral blood volume and hence ICP, but can cause accompanying reductions in global CBF, sometimes below ischaemic thresholds. Such ischaemia can be documented using jugular bulb oximetry, which may worsen outcome, specially when hyperventilation is prolonged or profound. The diffusible hydrogen ion acceptor, tetra-hydro-aminomethane (THAM), may restore ECF base levels and restore cerebrovascular CO_2 reactivity. While such an approach has been shown to reduce ICP and the need for intensification of ICP therapy after head injury, it does not alter outcome.

FLUID THERAPY AND FEEDING

Accurate fluid management may be complicated by continuing or concealed haemorrhage from associated extracranial trauma, but every effort must be made to restore normovolaemia and prevent hypotension. Fluid replacement should be guided by clinical and laboratory assessment of volume status and by invasive haemodynamic monitoring, but generally involves the administration of 30–40 ml/kg of maintenance fluid per day. The choice of hydration fluid is largely based on inconclusive results from animal data. Fluid flux across the normal BBB is governed by osmolarity rather than oncotic pressure. Consequently, hypotonic fluids are avoided and serum osmolality is maintained at high normal levels (290–300 mosm/l in our practice). Dextrose containing solutions are avoided since the residual free water after dextrose metabolism can worsen cerebral oedema, and because the associated elevations in blood sugar may worsen outcome.

Head-injured patients have high nutritional requirements and feeding should be instituted early (within 24 hours), aiming to replace 140% of resting metabolic expenditure (with 15% of calories supplied as protein) by the seventh day post trauma. Enteral feeding is associated with a lower incidence of hyperglycaemia and may have a protective effect against gastric ulceration. Impaired gastric emptying can be treated with prokinetic agents such as metoclopramide. In those who cannot be fed enterally, parenteral nutrition should be considered together with rigorous blood sugar control and some form of prophylaxis against gastric ulceration (H_2 antagonists or sucralfate).

HYPEROSMOLAR THERAPY

Mannitol (0.25–1 g/kg, usually as a 20% solution) has traditionally been used to elevate plasma osmolarity and reduce brain oedema in the setting of intracranial hypertension. Side effects can be minimised if its use is discontinued when it no longer produces significant ICP reduction, volume status is monitored and plasma osmolality is not allowed to rise above 320 mosm/l. Recent reports also highlight the successful use of 23.4% saline for treatment of intracranial hypertension refractory to mannitol.

SEDATION AND NEUROMUSCULAR BLOCKADE

Intravenous anaesthetic agents preserve pressure autoregulation and the cerebrovascular response to CO_2 (even at doses sufficient to abolish cortical activity) and decrease CBF, cerebral metabolism and ICP. While the reduction in flow and CBV are secondary to a reduction in metabolism, flow-metabolism coupling is not perfect, and the decrease in CBF may exceed the corresponding decrease in $CMRO_2$, with a widening of the cerebral arteriovenous oxygen content difference. Barbiturates have been largely replaced by other agents such as propofol, which possesses similar cerebrovascular effects but better pharmacokinetic profiles. However, propofol can induce hypotension and decrease CPP. Problems with lipid loading have been substantially ameliorated by the introduction of a 2% formulation of propofol. Midazolam is often used as an alternative in combination with fentanyl for sedating the patient with head injury. Opioids generally have negligible effects on CBF and $CMRO_2$. However, the newer synthetic opioids fentanyl, sufentanil and alfentanil, can increase ICP in patients with tumours and head trauma due to changes in $PaCO_2$ (in spontaneously breathing subjects) and reflex cerebral vasodilatation secondary to systemic hypotension. These changes can be avoided if blood pressure and ventilation are controlled.

Neuromuscular blockade in the head-injured patient receiving intensive care is currently the subject of much debate. Neuromuscular blockers can prevent rises in ICP produced by coughing and 'bucking on the tube'. However, overall outcome is not improved, perhaps because of increased respiratory complications and neuromyopathy remains a concern after long-term use (especially with the steroid-based agents). Atracurium is non-cumulative and has not been associated with myopathy, and theoretical concerns about the accumulation of laudanosine are not clinically relevant.

ANTIEPILEPTIC THERAPY

Post-traumatic seizures are commonest in patients with a GCS < 10, an intracranial haematoma, contusion, penetrating injury or depressed skull fractures. Such patients may form the most appropriate subgroup for acute (days to weeks) seizure prophylaxis following head injury.

CEREBRAL METABOLIC SUPPRESSANTS

Intravenous barbiturates have been used for ICP reduction for over 20 years. While they clearly result in cardiovascular depression, increased ICU stay and increases in pulmonary infections, it appears that they may benefit patients with intractable intracranial hypertension that responds to intravenous anaesthetics. They are administered as an intravenous infusion and titrated to produce burst suppression on EEG. The prolonged recovery associated with barbiturates suggests a role for other intravenous anaesthetics (etomidate and propofol) with more desirable pharmacokinetic profiles. However, the efficacy of these agents remains unproven, and they have their own drawbacks.

NOVEL NEUROPROTECTIVE INTERVENTIONS

While a variety of novel pharmacological neuroprotective agents are currently under investigation, none of the drugs that have been tested thus far in phase III trials have proved beneficial on an intention to treat basis.

HYPOTHERMIA

Mild to moderate hypothermia (33–36°C) has been shown to be neuroprotective in animal studies which demonstrated improved outcome from cerebral ischaemia with small (1–3°C) reductions in temperature. Three early clinical studies demonstrated benefit from moderate hypothermia in head injury, and interim results from a large ongoing outcome trial were encouraging, suggesting benefit in a subgroup of patients with GCS of 5–7. However, the study was terminated early on grounds of futility, with no clear benefit established. Initial post-hoc analysis suggests that younger patients with higher ICPs may benefit from hypothermia.

SEQUENTIAL ESCALATION VS TARGETED THERAPY FOR THE INTENSIVE CARE OF HEAD INJURY

It is clear that a diverse range of pathophysiological processes operate in acute head injury, and that there exist a wide range of therapeutic options, few of which have proven efficacy. One of two approaches may be used in the choice of therapy in such a setting. The first of these is to use a standard protocol in all patients, and introduce more intensive therapies in a sequence that is based either on intensity of intervention or on local experience and availability. Alternatively, individual therapies can be targeted at individual pathophysiological processes. Examples are the use of hyperventilation in the presence of hyperaemia, mannitol for vasogenic cerebral oedema or the use of blood pressure elevation in the presence of B waves.

In practice, many established head injury protocols represent a hybrid approach. Initial baseline monitoring and therapy are applied to all patients, and refractory problems are dealt with by therapy escalation, with the choice of intervention determined by clinical presentation and physiological monitoring. Often, interventions that are more difficult to implement or present significant risks (e.g. barbiturate coma) are used as a last resort. Figure 38.1 represents the ICP/CPP management protocol used in the Neurosciences Critical Care Unit at Addenbrooke's Hospital.

Addenbrooke's NCCU: ICP/CPP management algorithm

All patients with or at risk of intracranial hypertension *must* have invasive arterial monitoring, CVP line, ICP monitor and Rt SjO$_2$ catheter at admission to NCCU.

Efforts must be made to attach TCD and multimodality monitoring computer within the first six hours of NCCU stay.

Check whether the patient is or may be a candidate for research protocols.

Guidelines may be modified at the discretion of the consultant in charge.

Treatment grades III and IV should only be initiated after express approval of the Consultant in charge of NCCU.

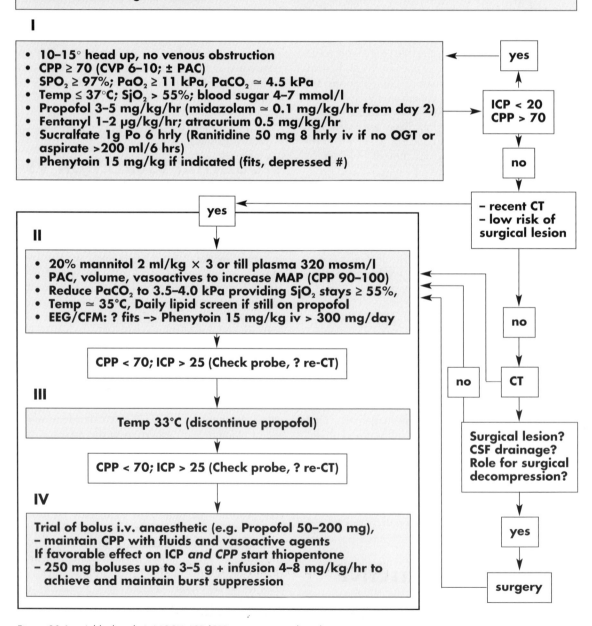

I

- 10–15° head up, no venous obstruction
- CPP ≥ 70 (CVP 6–10; ± PAC)
- SPO$_2$ ≥ 97%; PaO$_2$ ≥ 11 kPa, PaCO$_2$ ≈ 4.5 kPa
- Temp ≤ 37°C; SjO$_2$ > 55%; blood sugar 4–7 mmol/l
- Propofol 3–5 mg/kg/hr (midazolam ≈ 0.1 mg/kg/hr from day 2)
- Fentanyl 1–2 µg/kg/hr; atracurium 0.5 mg/kg/hr
- Sucralfate 1g Po 6 hrly (Ranitidine 50 mg 8 hrly iv if no OGT or aspirate >200 ml/6 hrs)
- Phenytoin 15 mg/kg if indicated (fits, depressed #)

yes

ICP < 20
CPP > 70

no

– recent CT
– low risk of surgical lesion

no

II

- 20% mannitol 2 ml/kg × 3 or till plasma 320 mosm/l
- PAC, volume, vasoactives to increase MAP (CPP 90–100)
- Reduce PaCO$_2$ to 3.5–4.0 kPa providing SjO$_2$ stays ≥ 55%,
- Temp ≈ 35°C, Daily lipid screen if still on propofol
- EEG/CFM: ? fits –> Phenytoin 15 mg/kg iv > 300 mg/day

yes

CPP < 70; ICP > 25 (Check probe, ? re-CT)

III

Temp 33°C (discontinue propofol)

CPP < 70; ICP > 25 (Check probe, ? re-CT)

no

CT

Surgical lesion?
CSF drainage?
Role for surgical decompression?

yes

IV

Trial of bolus i.v. anaesthetic (e.g. Propofol 50–200 mg),
– maintain CPP with fluids and vasoactive agents
If favorable effect on ICP *and CPP* start thiopentone
– 250 mg boluses up to 3–5 g + infusion 4–8 mg/kg/hr to achieve and maintain burst suppression

surgery

Figure 38.1   Addenbrooke's NCCU: ICP/CPP management algorithm

KEY POINTS

- The primary aim in the management of head-injured patients is the prevention of secondary brain injury.
- Hypoxia and hypotension must be avoided.
- There is regional heterogeneity in cerebral blood flow and metabolism after injury.
- Multimodal monitoring facilitates the early identification of secondary insults.
- Many centres target therapy to maintain CPP above 60–70 mmHg
- ICP should be kept below 25 mmHg.

RECOMMENDED READING

Brain Trauma Foundation. 1996. Guidelines for the management of severe head injury. Journal of Neurotrauma. 1996 13(11), 639–734

Jones PA, Andrews PJD, Midgley S et al. 1994 Measuring the burden of secondary insults in head injured patients during intensive care. Journal of Neurosurgical Anesthesiology 6, 4–14

Menon DK. 1999 Cerebral protection in severe brain injury: physiological determinants of outcome and their optimisation. British Medical Bulletin 55, 226–258

Menon DK, Summors AC. 1998 Neuroprotection (including hypothermia). Current Opinion in Anaesthesiology 11, 485–496

39

MANAGEMENT OF SUBARACHNOID HAEMORRHAGE

J. Ulatowski

INTRODUCTION

Although subarachnoid haemorrhage (SAH) is a relatively uncommon cause of stroke, it remains the most targeted stroke condition for diagnosis and treatment because of the possibility of a reasonable outcome with timely intervention. Urgency in diagnosis and treatment cannot be overstated as estimates for 30-day mortality reach 40%. This high-risk period also offers a window for successful therapies and critical care intervention (Table 27.1).

The critical care management of patients with SAH begins prior to hospitalisation. SAH presents suddenly, and a large number of patients succumb prior to hospital admission due to raised intracranial pressure causing syncope, respiratory depression and cardiac arrhythmia. Patients successfully arriving at emergency departments complain of severe headache ('worst headache of their life') with nausea, vomiting, photophobia and stiff neck (meningismus). Diagnosis begins with CT scan and, if negative, lumbar puncture performed meticulously to avoid traumatic puncture. Conventional angiography, CT angiography and MR angiography will confirm the presence of an aneurysm in most spontaneous SAH cases. Patients with normal angiograms have a repeat study prior to diagnosing non-aneurysmal SAH.

Initial treatment involves stabilisation of vital signs (airway, breathing, circulation) and preventing sequelae of SAH such as rebleeding, hydrocephalus, seizures and vasospasm in the period before and after surgical or angiographic-guided ablation of the aneurysm.

Table 27.1 Critical care intervention after SAH

Condition	Diagnosis	Treatment
Preoperative		
Syncope	CT scan	
	intracerebral clot	Evacuation, treat oedema
	hydrocephalus	ventricular CSF drainage
Cardiovascular		
Arrhythmia	ECG	Anti-arrhythmic, correct electrolytes
Hypotension	Myocardial enzymes, ECG, ECHO	Intravascular volume and inotropic support
Hypertension	ECG, assess blood volume	Prevent rebleeding, anti-hypertensive therapy, sedation, pain control
Pulmonary		
Pneumonia	Chest X-ray	Oxygen, antibiotics, intubation, mechanical ventilation
Pulmonary oedema	Chest X-ray	Oxygen, intubation, PEEP, mechanical ventilation
Seizures	Electroencephalogram (EEG)	Anticonvulsants
Postoperative		
Delayed cerebral ischaemia (vasospasm)	CT scan	
	Surgical retraction injury	Maintain MAP, treat oedema
	Hydrocephalus	CSF drainage
	No lesion	Calcium channel blockers,
	TCD blood flow velocity increases at stenosis	HHH therapy, angioplasty, papaverine infusion
Congestive heart failure and pulmonary oedema	ECG, ECHO, chest X-ray Pulmonary artery catheter	Diuresis, inotropic support, PEEP
Electrolyte disturbance (hyponatremia)	Blood sampling	Repletion
Cerebral salt wasting	Assess volume	Sodium & blood volume repletion
Syndrome of inappropriate ADH secretion	Plasma & urine osmolality	Free water intake restriction
Nutrition	Caloric intake	Enteral, parenteral supplementation, gastrostomy
Prolonged ventilation	Weaning trials, assess airway competency	Trial of extubation, tracheostomy
Deep venous thrombosis	Doppler ultrasound of extremities	Heparin, coumadin, vena cava filter

For further information on the presentation and natural history of SAH see Chapter 13.

INTENSIVE CARE MANAGEMENT

Patients presenting with significant neurological deficit from SAH usually have substantial parenchymal injury due to intracerebral extension of clot, mass effect, hydrocephalus (raised ICP) and seizures. Decreased level of consciousness and arrhythmia must be treated to prevent aspiration pneumonia or respiratory failure and haemodynamic decline while surgical options (evacuation of clot or external ventricular drainage of CSF) are addressed. This simultaneous team effort involving intensive care physicians, neurologists and neurosurgeons, requires coordination that usually occurs in the ICU.

BLOOD PRESSURE CONTROL

Preoperative ICU management concentrates on normalisation of blood pressure to reduce the risk of rebleeding. Caution is advised not to reduce MAP quickly. Blood pressure management should be guided by changes in neurological exam (ischaemic symptoms), maintaining CPP between 70 and 90 mmHg and/or ensuring adequate cerebral perfusion by measuring cerebral oximetry with a jugular venous catheter, indwelling oximetric probe or transcutaneous oximetry for patients in stupor or coma. Blood pressure should be reduced (SBP < 180 mmHg) within the first 2 hours followed by normalisation of BP if tolerated within 4–8 hours. Calcium channel blockers used for neuroprotection (nimodipine, nicardipine) may be supplemented with other drugs such as labetalol or captopril. Direct-acting vasodilators (nitrates, hydralazine) may increase cerebral blood volume causing raised ICP and are a last resort.

Preventive measures to reduce elevations in blood pressure are also invoked. This may include keeping the patient sedated and analgesed using short-acting sedative and narcotic medications. Bedside activities are kept to a minimum to prevent agitation. For good grade patients (Hunt and Hess grade I–II), invasive cardiovascular monitoring and other testing is postponed until the time of surgery. The diet is kept simple and avoids caffeinated products. A laxative may be used to prevent straining during bowel movements. Finally, the patient should be reassured that they are in a safe environment and that there is a therapy for their disease. Patients with grades III–V

require intubation, supported ventilation and sedation with full monitoring.

CARDIAC FUNCTION

Cardiac arrhythmias and changes in cardiac function occur in approximately 50% of patients. The most common are electrocardiographic abnormalities, many of which are non-specific (sinus tachycardia, T-wave inversion, U waves, QT interval prolongation). However, others may be more ominous including variable states of heart block, premature atrial and ventricular ectopy that may lead to tachycardia, ST segment depression, and elevated cardiac enzymes associated with echocardiographic ventricular wall abnormalities. Most of these occur immediately after SAH and are probably due to transient catecholamine release. As a result, beta blocker medications are a first choice for treating cardiac complications in these patients. Further cardiovascular testing and therapy may be necessary to rule out ongoing myocardial ischaemia prior to surgery.

SEIZURES

Seizures can occur at various points after SAH, but are generally thought to be infrequent. Abnormal motor posturing is witnessed with onset of SAH. This may be as a result of overall depression of the nervous system (herniation) or generalised seizures, both due to transient ischaemia caused by the initial increase in ICP. Seizures in the first 1–2 weeks after aneurysm rupture and surgery occur in approximately 1–3% of patients. Prophylactic phenytoin treatment is routine in many centres during the period prior to aneurysm clipping and, although still controversial, proponents argue that seizure prevention lessens the chance of rebleeding, hypertension and transient hypoxaemia. Prolonged postoperative seizure prophylaxis has no proven benefit, therefore anticonvulsants are most commonly used during the first 7–14 days after SAH and only continued in patients with witnessed seizures. Further therapy is guided by improvement in neurological status and EEG studies.

HYDROCEPHALUS

Hydrocephalus occurs in two forms after SAH. **Communicating hydrocephalus** is due to blockage of CSF outflow at the arachnoid granulations. **Non-communicating (obstructive) hydrocephalus** is due to the obstruction of CSF outflow from the ventricular system either by large clots leading to external compression or to bleeding into the ventricles. Intraventricular haemorrhage is more common with anterior cerebral artery and vertebrobasilar artery aneurysms. Hydrocephalus can be part of the initial presentation of SAH or can occur at any time in the postoperative period presenting as a decline in level of consciousness. Early after SAH, hydrocephalus can make the initial neurological exam appear more grave than actual parenchymal damage would indicate. Later it can mimic global ischaemia from vasospasm.

Hydrocephalus (communicating and non-communicating) is usually treated with external ventricular drainage using a temporary indwelling catheter, which also allows measurement of ICP. CSF can be drained to reduce pressure and maintain adequate cerebral perfusion pressure. Slow drainage of CSF in patients with untreated aneurysms is recommended to avoid rapid changes in transmural forces across the aneurysm wall or settling of the brain thereby compressing the aneurysm and leading to rebleeding. Most patients with obstructive hydrocephalus eventually clear the blood from the ventricular system but may have persistent hydrocephalus due to continued interruption of CSF outflow at the arachnoid granulations. Should this condition become more chronic, the intraventricular catheter can be changed to lessen risk of infection or substituted with lumbar CSF drainage. Alternatively, frequent spinal taps are used for communicating hydrocephalus before determining the need for permanent shunting.

PULMONARY COMPLICATIONS

Pulmonary complications are more rare after SAH; however, they account for 50% of the medical mortality. Pneumonia occurs due to aspiration in patients with a decreased level of consciousness with or without an endotracheal tube. Neurogenic pulmonary oedema can occur in approximately 2% of patients who present in coma. Treatment includes endotracheal intubation and mechanical ventilatory support using positive end-expiratory pressure and supplemental oxygen. A pulmonary artery catheter is sometimes inserted to differentiate cardiac from pulmonary oedema, both of which can occur after SAH.

GENERAL CARE

General medical care includes attention to electrolyte disturbances (sodium and potassium predominantly),

prophylactic gastrointestinal antacid therapy (especially in patients treated with steroids), pre-emptive treatment of constipation that can occur in bedridden patients, facilitated early nutrition and prevention of deep venous thrombosis and bedsores in immobilised patients. Normothermia should be maintained, by active cooling if necessary.

SURGERY

Timing of surgery can either be early (1–3 days after SAH) or late (10–14 days). Early surgery reduces the risk of rebleed, and early removal of the blood clot may reduce the risk of vasospasm. Late surgery is technically easier. Although there is still debate as to optimal timing, in many institutions surgery is performed within 4 days after SAH.

Onset of global or focal ischaemia due to cerebral vasospasm is delayed ranging from day 4 to day 21 following aneurysmal rupture, with a peak incidence on days 5–10. Best evidence supports the presence of blood products around the large arteries at the base of the brain as a cause for the segmental narrowing of the blood vessels. Not surprisingly the best predictor of vasospasm is the amount of the subarachnoid blood detected by CT scan. Angiographic studies have demonstrated cerebral vasospasm to occur in 60–75% of patients. However, with current therapy, one-third of SAH patients develop clinical symptoms of delayed ischaemia. Serial neurological examinations supplemented by TCD is used for monitoring onset of vasospasm. Vasospasm is frequently treated prophylactically with calcium channel blockers (nimodipine or nicardipine). Angiographic studies have not confirmed reversal of vasospasm in larger arteries implying that the effect is of calcium channel blockers on small distal vessels or a direct neuroprotective effect in brain tissue. This treatment continues for 21 days.

Hypervolaemia, hypertension, haemodilution (HHH) therapy is thought to improve neurological status and decrease the incidence of neurological deficits and death due to vasospasm. However, evidence of long term benefit is scarce and there is the potential for many complications. Increasing blood volume with crystalloid or colloid solutions to achieve a haematocrit of 30% after aneurysmal repair facilitates haemodilution and spontaneous hypertension. The combination of a reduced blood viscosity and higher blood pressure proximal to the stenosis is believed to increase cerebral perfusion. If symptoms persist with only moderate increases in blood pressure (MAP 90–110 mmHg) further haemodynamic augmentation with inotropes (e.g. dopamine 2.5–15 μg/kg/min) or vasoconstrictors is commenced and guided by use of a pulmonary artery catheter. Care must be taken to maintain systolic blood pressure below 150 mmHg in patients with unclipped aneurysms. If neurological improvement is not achieved using this therapy, more aggressive treatments are tried (see below).

Balloon angioplasty to directly dilate accessible vessels has shown good results in cases of refractory vasospasm. Mechanical dilatation of the intracerebral vessels has been shown to increase distal perfusion and the effect appears to be long-lasting. Intra-arterial injection of papavarine, (a vasodilator), alone or in addition to angioplasty, is also believed to improve brain blood flow. The effect of these two therapies may be delayed as late as 12–36 hours. Lack of controlled trials demonstrating effect on outcome, as well as limited technical expertise, has relegated this treatment to large academic centres with ongoing studies.

Improvements in neurological symptoms and normalisation of TCD velocities guide the intensity and duration of therapy for cerebral vasospasm. HHH therapy is weaned slowly over hours to days while observing for recurrence of symptoms. Calcium channel blockers are stopped after 3 weeks of therapy and replaced by long-term anti-hypertensive therapy if indicated. If prolonged intubation (beyond 10 days) is anticipated, an elective tracheostomy is performed. Patients unable to maintain nutritional intake sufficient to sustain recovery undergo gastrostomy tube placement. Once these and other general medical conditions have been stabilised, patients can be transferred from intensive care.

KEY POINTS

- Intensive care management of patients with SAH begins early in the course of therapy and continues throughout a variable period
- Hydrocephalus and vasospasm may complicate recovery despite successful ablation of the aneurysm
- Systemic complications need to be treated pre-operatively
- Vasospasm can be treated with HHH therapy in ICU, or angiographically using papaverine or balloon angioplasty.

REFERENCES

1. Sacco RL et al. Subarachnoid and intracerebral hemorrhage: natural history, prognosis, and precursive factors in the Framingham Study. Neurology 1984; 34(7): 847–854
2. Rinkel GJ, Djibuti M and van Gijn J. Prevalence and risk of rupture of intracranial aneurysms: a systematic review. Stroke 1998; 29(1): 251–256
3. Mayberg MR et al. Guidelines for the management of aneurysmal subarachnoid hemorrhage. A statement for healthcare professionals from a special writing group of the Stroke Council, American Heart Association. Stroke 1994; 25(11): 2315–2328
4. Weir B. Subarachnoid hemorrhage: causes and cures. CNS: Contemporary Neurology Series, Vol. 52. Oxford University Press, New York, 1998
5. Hunt WE, Hess RM. Surgical risk as related to time of intervention in the repair of intracranial aneurysms. J Neurosurg 1968; 28(1): 14–20
6. Solenski NJ et al. Medical complications of aneurysmal subarachnoid hemorrhage: a report of the multicenter, cooperative aneurysm study. Participants of the Multicenter Cooperative Aneurysm Study [see comments]. Crit Care Med 1995; 23(6): 1007–1017
7. McKhann GM II, Le Roux PD. Perioperative and intensive care unit care of patients with aneurysmal subarachnoid hemorrhage. Neurosurg Clin N Am 1998; 9(3): 595–613

40

NEUROPROTECTION IN ICU

A. Summors, P. Doyle, A.K. Gupta

PRINCIPLES OF NEUROPROTECTION

Current strategies for brain protection focus around prevention of secondary injury (Table 40.1).

The pathophysiological mechanisms of secondary injury are complex, but have common manifestations such as reduced CBF or raised ICP. Laboratory studies have identified many potential therapeutic interventions that might have clinical application following brain injury (e.g. antagonism of inflammatory mediators, hypothermia, gene therapy and neural transplantation). Many of these therapies have progressed into completed clinical trials, and others have been prematurely terminated or are in various phases of testing. The results of completed phase III drug trials have been generally disappointing compared with the success in animal laboratory studies, with few, if any, drug treatments proving to improve outcome.

Neuroprotection strategies can be categorised into optimising physiology, pharmacological methods and non-pharmacological interventions.

OPTIMISING PHYSIOLOGY

Maintenance of CBF and oxygenation

Chestnut et al demonstrated that hypotension (systolic blood pressure < 90 mmHg) and hypoxia (PaO_2 < 60 mmHg) after head injury were independent predictors of poor outcome.[1] Careful fluid management and the use of inotropes should ensure an adequate CPP. Adequate sedation reduces agitation and may help control ICP (see Chapter 44). Low dose propofol has been shown to be superior to morphine at controlling ICP but gives no improvement in neurological outcome.

Hyperventilation

Hypocapnia causes cerebral vasoconstriction thereby reducing CBV and hence ICP. Whilst hyperventilation may help reduce ICP, two issues need consideration:

1. Hyperventilation causes a reduction in both global and regional CBF which may fall below ischaemic thresholds. This is most commonly detected by jugular bulb desaturation (< 50%) and is associated with a poor outcome. In our unit, $PaCO_2$ is kept above 4 kPa in an attempt to maintain an adequate CBF.
2. The effects of hyperventilation on ICP are often temporary due to pH compensation in the brain and CSF, and may lead to a rebound rise in cerebral blood volume and ICP when arterial CO_2 is normalised.

Normoglycaemia

The brain is dependent on exogenous glucose for its cellular energy requirements. During ischaemia, anaerobic glycolysis produces lactate which is regarded as neurotoxic *per se*. The amount of lactate formed depends on the duration and severity of ischaemia and the pre-existing stores of glucose and glycogen. The higher the concentration of glucose, the more lactate is formed, thereby aggravating brain injury. Tight glucose control is essential with routine measurement of blood glucose levels and avoidance of glucose containing fluids. Insulin infusions may be needed.

PHARMACOLOGICAL THERAPY

Anaesthetic agents

The primary mechanism by which the anaesthetic agents confer neuroprotective effects involves a

---

Table 40.1 Mechanisms of brain injury. Initial event: trauma, ischaemia

Primary	Secondary	Systemic insult
• Tissue destruction	• Pressure effects	• Hypoxaemia
• Haemorrhage	• Hydrocephalus	• Hypotension
• Pressure effects	• Herniation	• Hypercarbia
• Diffuse axonal injury	• Vasospasm	• Excessive hypocarbia
	• Reduced metabolic rate	• Hyperthermia
	• Impaired autoregulation	• Anaemia
	• Secondary hyperaemia	• Electrolyte disturbance
	• Oedema	• Hyperglycaemia

decrease in $CMRO_2$ and reduction in the energy used for synaptic transmission. Other mechanisms are given in Table 40.2.

Barbiturates have been found to be particularly useful in focal ischaemia, although there is little evidence of neuroprotective effects in global ischaemia (e.g. post cardiac arrest). Thiopentone has proven useful in status epilepticus and during periods of ischaemia in refractory intracranial hypertension. It may also allow prolonged temporary clipping during aneurysm surgery, although there is no evidence of improvement in overall outcome. Thiopentone should be titrated to EEG burst suppression (250 mg bolus up to 3–5 g, followed by infusions of 4–8 mg/kg/h) in refractory intracranial hypertension, and care should be taken to maintain CPP.

There is currently no good evidence demonstrating the clinical benefit of other intravenous anaesthetic agents such as propofol, etomidate, ketamine, opioids or benzodiazepines as neuroprotective agents.

Although the volatile anaesthetic agents reduce $CMRO_2$, it appears that this only extends to cortical activity and not membrane/organelle function. This provides cerebral protection for only a short time and is of no proven clinical benefit.

Steroids

Although there is evidence of benefit in the early administration of high dose methylprednisolone in spinal cord injury (see Chapter 35), there is no such evidence of benefit from corticosteroids in the intensive care management of head injury.

Table 40.2 Neuroprotection mechanisms of anaesthetic agents

- Reduction in synaptic transmission
- Reduction in Calcium influx
- Na^+ channel blockade
- Membrane stabilisation
- Improvement in distribution of regional blood flow
- Suppression of cortical EEG activity
- Reduction in cerebral oedema
- Free radical scavenging
- Potentiate γ-aminobutyrate activity
- Alteration of free fatty acid metabolism
- Suppression of catecholamine-induced hyperactivity
- Reduction in CSF secretion
- Deafferentation and immobilisation
- Uptake of glutamate in synapses

Calcium channel blockade

Intracellular calcium accumulation is thought to be a major cause of cellular injury during ischaemia due to a disruption of certain subtypes of voltage gated Ca^{++} channels (i.e. N, Q and P) regulating Ca^{++} influx into cells and mitochondria. Whilst the exact protective mechanism of calcium channel blockers is still not fully understood, it is probable that they reduce the influx of Ca^{++} across plasma and mitochondrial membranes.

Calcium channel antagonists (e.g. nimodipine) provide protection following SAH. The mechanism of protection is not by prevention of vasospasm as initially thought, but probably by direct cytoprotective effects. There is no good evidence of benefit of these agents in traumatic brain injury.

Sodium channel blockade

Anticonvulsants such as phenytoin (and its prodrug fosphenytoin), lamotrigine, lubeluzole and riluzole act by Na^+ channel blockade, decreasing neuronal transmission and energy requirements for neuronal transmission. Attenuation of release of the excitatory amino acid glutamate also occurs. All have been proven effective experimentally in providing neuroprotection, but have been disappointing in the clinical setting.

Other sodium channel blockers that have shown promise in vitro are the local anaesthetic agents, QX314 and QX222 and a new opioid with Na^+ blocking properties, called Enadoline. These are still under investigation.

Excitatory amino acid (EAA) antagonists

Glutamate and aspartate are the major EAAs present during ischaemia and concentrations of these EAAs are vastly increased in the extracellular space. This causes a surge of neuronal activity mediated by four different types of glutamate receptor – NMDA, AMPA (a-amino-3-hydroxy-5-methyl-4-isoxazole propionic acid), Kainate, metabotropic receptors. The NMDA receptor is the major route allowing Ca^{2+} into the cytosol (a process normally blocked by Mg^{2+}). Excessive activation of these receptors can trigger a huge influx of Ca^{2+} intracellularly with concomitant increases in permeability for other ions.

The neuroprotective effects of EAA antagonists have been demonstrated in animal models of head injury. Selfotel was a recent compound, which like others showed promise in animal models but did not progress into clinical use.

NSAIDS

Prostoglandin inhibitors such as indomethacin cause cerebral vasoconstriction by reducing prostacyclin synthesis, thus reducing ICP, but a rebound phenomena may be seen if stopped suddenly.

Other novel therapies

No efficacy has been demonstrated in multicentred trials with antioxidants; (tirilazad mesylate, pegorgotein) or Deltibant (a bradykinin antagonist).

A number of different successful experimental therapies (Table 40.3) are awaiting clinical trials.

NON-PHARMACOLOGICAL METHODS

Hypothermia

Moderate hypothermia (32–33°C) improves outcome in animal models by reducing:

1. $CMRO_2$
2. Neurotransmitter synthesis, release and reuptake
3. Frequency of energy depleting ischaemic depolarisations
4. Free radical production
5. Intracranial hypertension.

In addition there is better preservation of the blood–brain barrier, cytoskeleton integrity and modulation of apoptotic gene expression.

In the clinical setting, the debate over efficacy continues. The Multicentre National Hypothermia Trial has been stopped prematurely although no results have been published as yet. However, Marion et al, in a large single-centred study of head injured patients demonstrated an improvement in outcome after hypothermia (33°C) at 3 and 6 months in a subgroup of patients with GCS 5–7.[2]

Intraoperative hypothermia during aneurysm surgery is currently being investigated in a large multicentred randomised trial which has recently commenced.

The success of hypothermic neuroprotection in models of head injury may simply be the avoidance of *hyperthermia* in the injured brain, which is detrimental to outcome. Ischaemic brain is warmer than systemic temperature, and maintenance of normothermia is important – the best means of achieving this is forced convective cooling. Pharmacological methods for temperature reduction have unsustained effects.

HHH THERAPY (HYPERTENSION, HYPERVOLAEMIA, HAEMODILUTION)

HHH therapy gives short-term improvement in neurological function for vasopasm following SAH. Evidence of long-term benefit is scarce and there is the potential for many complications (Table 40.4). MAP is increased to a level consistent with clinical improvement or to a systolic maximum of 140–150 mmHg for unclipped aneurysms, or 180–200 mmHg for secured aneurysms. This can be achieved with hypervolaemia with intravenous crystalloid or colloid solutions to a PAWP of 16–18 mmHg, followed by the addition of inotropes or vasoconstrictors. Haemodilution to a haematocrit of approximately 30% ensures maximal O_2 delivery to cerebral tissue.

KEY POINTS

- Neuroprotection aims to prevent secondary brain injury
- Individual therapy can be targeted with modern imaging techniques and cerebral monitoring
- Guiding principles are optimal physiology augmented with pharmacological and non-pharmacological methods

---

Table 40.3 Novel neuroprotective mechanisms and targets

Nitric oxide	Variable success with both inhibitors of NO synthesis and NO donors
Calpain	Protease acting on structural and regulatory proteins involved in injury; inhibition provides protection
Immunophilins	e.g. Cyclosporin A & FK506 inhibit calcineurin and NO synthesis, modulate neurotransmitter release & cytosolic Ca^{++} increases and mediate nerve growth
PARP/Caspases	(Poly (ADP-ribose) polymerase) a DNA repair enzyme activated on injury and depleting energy stores at a time when they are critical; Caspases involved in PARP activation and inhibition is protective
Matrix metalloproteases	Released in injury and disrupts BBB; inhibition is protective
Adenosine	Improves microvascular flow, inhibits platelet aggregation, role in ischaemic preconditioning; but action on some receptor subtypes may worsen injury

TABLE 40.4 Potential complications following HHH therapy

Cerebral	Vasogenic oedema
	Haemorrhage
	Aneurysmal rupture
	Increased ICP
Pulmonary	Oedema
Cardiac	Ischaemia/infarction

- Success of pharmacological therapies in animal models has not translated into drugs which improve outcome in clinical practice
- The beneficial effects of moderate hypothermia in acute brain injury is still under debate
- Methylprednisolone administered soon after spinal cord injury is of proven benefit.

REFERENCES

1. Chesnut RM, Marshall SB, Piek J et al. Early and late systemic hypotension as a frequent and fundamental source of cerebral ischaemia following severe brain injury in the Traumatic Coma Data Bank. Acta Neurochirurgica 1993; 59(suppl): 121–125

2. Marion DW, Penrod LE, Kelsey SF et al. Treatment of traumatic brain injury with moderate hypothermia. N Engl J Med 1997; 336: 540–546

FURTHER READING

Menon DK, Summors AC. Neuroprotection (including hypothermia). Cur Opin Anethesiol 1998; 11: 485–496

Doyle PW, Gupta AK. Mechanisms of injury and cerebral protection. In: Matta B, Menon DK, Turner JM (eds) Textbook of neuroanaesthesia and critical care. Greenwich Medical Media, London 2000, pp. 35–51

Bracken MB, Shepard MJ, Collins WF et al. A randomized controlled trial of methyl-prednisolone or naloxone in the treatment of acute spinal cord injury. N Engl J Med 1990; 322: 1405

Eker C, Asgeirsson B, Grande PO, Schalen W, Nordstrom CH. Improved outcome after severe head injury with a new therapy based on principles for brain volume regulation and preserved microcirculation. Crit Care Med 1998; 26: 1881–1886

Doppenberg EMR, Bullock R. Clinical neuroprotection trials in severe traumatic brain injury: Lessons from previous studies. J Neurotrauma 1997; 14(2): 71–80

41

INOTROPES IN
NEURO-CRITICAL CARE

R. Shankar

INTRODUCTION

Prevention of secondary brain damage is the primary aim of the intensive care management of the head injured patient. Many studies have demonstrated that increasing CPP improves the outcome in acute brain injury.

Cerebral perfusion may be increased by:

- reducing ICP
- increasing MAP
- increasing CBF by injection of papaverine (for vasospasm after sub-arachnoid haemorrhage) or balloon angioplasty of spastic vessels

THEORIES OF HEAD INJURY MANAGEMENT

There are two approaches to CPP management in head injury. The first preserves a CPP of >70 mmHg (controlled hypertension concept), and the other suggests reducing the CPP in an attempt to prevent oedema (Lund concept).

INDICATIONS FOR INOTROPE SUPPORT

- Maintain CPP in the presence of a raised ICP
- To enhance blood flow across spastic blood vessels associated with subarachnoid haemorrhage
- Manipulation of autoregulation
- Maintain cardiac output and haemodynamic support.

PHARMACOLOGY

Catecholamines

Dopamine, norepinephrine, epinephrine and phenylephrine are the agents frequently used in the intensive care unit. The physiological effects are due to dose-dependent stimulation of DA, α and β receptors. Side-effects are an extension of these physiological effects.

Receptors undergo down-regulation when exposed to a continuous infusion of large doses of catecholamines and frequent adjustments in infusion rate are required to maintain the haemodynamic targets.

Dopamine

Dopamine is a naturally occurring catecholamine, and a precursor of epinephrine and norepinephrine. The haemodynamic effects and side-effects vary according to the type of receptor stimulated, which in turn depends on the rate of infusion (Table 41.1).

Table 41.1 Physiological effects of dopamine infusion

Dose (μg/kg/min)	Predominant Receptors stimulated	Clinical effects
Up to 5	Dopamine	Renal and mesenteric vasodilatation causing hypotension Increased urine output
5–15	β_1	Positive cardiac inotropy and chronotropy
>15	α_1	Peripheral vasoconstriction

Epinephrine

Epinephrine stimulates β receptors at low doses leading to tachycardia and increased cardiac index. α receptors are stimulated at higher doses leading to systolic hypertension, but the diastolic pressures may remain low with the MAP remaining the same or decreasing slightly. It is for this reason that epinephrine is not the favoured inotrope to drive the MAP in the neuro-intensive care setting. The initial infusion rate is 0.05 μg/kg/min.

Norepinephrine

Norepinephrine stimulates α receptors predominantly although there are some β effects. The haemodynamic effects are systolic and diastolic hypertension with an increase in MAP and possibly reflex bradycardia. The initial infusion rate is 0.05 μg/kg/min. Although CPP is increased, the effect on CBF is still undetermined as cerebral vasoconstriction may also occur.

Side-effects of inotropes

Tachyarrhythmias, hypoperfusion of organs, myocardial ischaemic hyperglycaemia, hypophosphataemia and hypocalcaemia may all be seen.

CLINICAL APPLICATIONS

Continuous monitoring of MAP, ICP, and CPP helps to optimise CBF and improve the outcome of patients with acute brain injury.

The arterial transducer should be zeroed to the level of the foramen of Monroe. The external landmark is the junction between the middle and posterior thirds of a line joining the lateral angle of the eye to the tragus. The difference between the MAP measured at the level of the heart and the foramen of Monroe is directly proportional to the height of the patient and the degree of elevation of the head. In a critical state of reduced intracranial compliance, even a small differences become clinically significant.

Maintainance of cerebral blood flow

Inotropes should be titrated to maintain a CPP of approximately 70 mmHg. Driving the CPP over 105 mmHg increases the formation of oedema in areas of contusion and increases the risk of myocardial ischaemia. It is imperative to optimise intravascular volume prior to commencement of inotropes.

In our institution, the first choice inotrope is often dopamine with infusion rates of 2–10 μg/kg/min, where β effects predominate. In this situation dopamine is considered to have a more specific effect on the force of contraction than on the heart rate, although tachycardia and arrhythmias may be a problem especially if the intravascular compartment is contracted.

If dopamine fails to improve the CPP, or if side-effects are problematic, an infusion of norepinephrine should be commenced in an effort to maintain an adequate CPP. Floating a pulmonary artery catheter at this juncture will guide fluid management and help assess the haemodynamic effects of norepinepherine.

Enhancement of blood flow across spastic blood vessels

Inotropes are used to increase the MAP as part of HHH therapy. The aim is to increase the MAP sufficiently to reverse the neurological deficit, usually with MAP ranging between 100 and 110 mmHg.

Manipulation of autoregulation

A fall in the MAP will reduce the CPP, if the ICP is stable. This fall in CPP results in cerebral vaso-dilatation in an attempt to improve CBF and in turn this leads to an increased CBV and increased ICP in a brain with poor intracranial compliance. This cycle of events is represented in Figure 41.1. In such a situation, vasopressors may be used to increase the MAP to break the cycle and reduce the ICP.

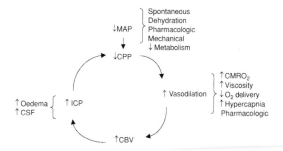

Figure 41.1   Cycle of events associated with a fall in MAP. Reproduced with permission from Rosner et al.

KEY POINTS

- Inotropes are used to enhance CPP and CBF
- Optimisation of intra-vascular volume prior to use of inotropes is mandatory
- The ideal agent to improve CPP is still undetermined.

FURTHER READING

Rosner MJ et al. 1995 Cerebral perfusion pressure: management protocol and clinical results. J Neurosurgery, 83(6): 949–962.

Chestnut RM. 1998 Hyperventilation versus cerebral perfusion pressure management, time to change the question. [editorial; comment]. Crit Care Med 26(2): 210–212.

Grande PO. 1997 Aspects on the cerebral perfusion pressure during therapy of a traumatic head injury. Acta Anaesthesiol Scand Suppl 110: 36–40.

Nates JL. 1997 Cerebral perfusion pressure monitoring alert! Crit Care Med 25(5): 895–896.

42

ELECTROLYTE DISORDERS IN THE NEUROINTENSIVE CARE UNIT

J. Ulatowski

INTRODUCTION

Electrolyte imbalance can lead to a wide variety of symptoms affecting many cell types and organs. These disturbances can occur because of reduced or excess intake of electrolytes, diseases of the endocrine organs controlling electrolyte concentrations (absorption and excretion), or iatrogenic changes in the fluid and electrolyte balance (such as administration of incorrect electrolyte concentrations or inappropriate fluid volume). Furthermore, endocrine function may be disturbed and fluid and electrolyte concentrations may be deregulated as part of multi-system failure in ICU patients. Finally, certain diseases involve or require treatment (such as massive fluid resuscitation) which significantly affects the fluid balance within the body.

Fluid and electrolyte imbalances can lead to a variety of symptoms in the intensive care population. Disturbances of calcium, magnesium and potassium can lead to cardiovascular changes including hypotension and arrhythmia. Disturbances in these same electrolytes can cause irritability in nerve and muscle function. Hypophosphataemia can lead to muscle weakness of the limbs and diaphragm. However, the most common conditions seen in the neurointensive care unit involve disturbances in sodium and water balance.

SODIUM AND WATER BALANCE

The measured concentration of any ion must be interpreted in the context of circulating or total body fluid volume because ion concentrations can be affected by changes in the solute (e.g. sodium) or the solvent (i.e. water).

Although sodium and water homeostasis is controlled by separate hormone systems within the body, the trigger for initiating changes in sodium and water control may be shared. For instance, significant intravascular volume loss will stimulate both sodium and water retention and is initiated through a baroreceptor response in the atria of the heart and the aorta. The effector of sodium retention is mainly through the action of aldosterone via the renin–angiotensin system. Water retention is controlled by antidiuretic hormone (ADH) secreted from the neurohypophysis. In addition to responding to gross changes in intravascular volume there are more delicate controls to fine-tune sodium and water balance. Osmo-receptors in the periventricular organs of the brain are extremely sensitive to small changes in serum osmolality and result in more minor secretion of ADH.

PATHOLOGY

Hypernatraemia

The most common causes of hypernatraemia in the neurointensive care unit are neurogenic diabetes insipidus (DI), mannitol induced diuresis, water dehydration from lack of intake in neurologically impaired individuals and, more recently, the administration of large volumes of hypertonic saline for the treatment of cerebral oedema and raised intracranial pressure. Acute elevations in sodium concentration due to excessive free water losses which occur rapidly from DI are corrected by the administration of hypotonic fluids (e.g. 0.45% saline) and intravenous vasopressin (0.5–1 μg desmopressin). More chronic hypernatraemic states due to prolonged dehydration or administration of hypertonic saline infusions over periods of days should be reversed more slowly. Brain cells exposed to chronically high concentrations of sodium will form what has been termed 'ideogenic osmoles'. These osmoles act as a strong osmotic force drawing water into brain cells when plasma fluid suddenly becomes isotonic. Brain oedema can ensue.

Diagnosing the cause of hypernatraemia is not difficult if an evaluation of intravascular volume can be performed. Dehydration, and DI result in decreases in plasma volume and can be diagnosed by decreased skin turgor, orthostatic blood pressure changes and reduction in central venous pressure. A low urine osmolality and high plasma osmolality is seen in DI (Fig. 42.1), with a urine specific gravity of < 1.005, and high urine output. In neurologically impaired individuals who cannot maintain intake of water,

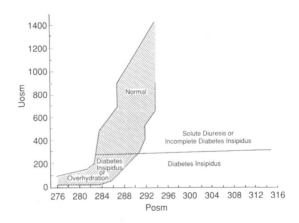

Figure 42.1   Relationship of plasma to urinary osmolality under normal and polyuric conditions. Adapted from Moses, with permission from the publisher

hypotonic intravenous fluids are required to maintain sodium and vascular volume near normal. Hypernatraemia due to the administration of hypertonic fluids usually is not associated with intravascular volume depletion. Correction will usually occur slowly by administration of isotonic fluids.

Hyponatraemia

Hyponatraemia can be caused by a relative increased retention of water, or as a result of relative loss of sodium. Long-term anticonvulsant intake (e.g. carbamazepine) should also be considered. Cerebral salt wasting is a syndrome commonly associated with neurological disease where natriuretic compounds secreted from the atria of the heart, and possibly the periventricular organs in the brain, are responsible for inducing sodium loss in the kidney. Hyponatraemia seen in these conditions may be potentiated by an appropriate ADH secretion in an attempt to compensate for hypovolaemia. Treatment of hyponatraemia in the face of hypovolaemia is by repletion with isotonic or hypertonic solutions depending on severity ($\leq$ 125 mmol/L). Rapid correction of hyponatraemia ($>$ 3 mmol/h) may result in a demyelinating state called central pontine myelinolysis.

The syndrome of inappropriate ADH secretion (SIADH) occurs when ADH is secreted without an osmotic trigger. Neurological disease is a common cause of SIADH, because the osmostatic cells in the brain are involved with the offending process. Patients with SIADH have normal intravascular volume and the urine is less than maximally dilute given the degree of relative water excess within the plasma. In order to make a diagnosis of SIADH, the patient must be normovolemic and have no evidence of adrenal or thyroid insufficiency, or excessive renal losses of fluid. Treatment is to restrict free water administration, and in severe states with addition of furosemide to induce a diuresis greater than natriuresis or democlocycline which impairs the effect of ADH on the kidney.

OTHER ELECTROLYTES

Hyperkalaemia

Hyperkalaemia from iatrogenic administration, or reduced excretion of potassium due to renal failure can cause life-threatening arrhythmia. Particular to the neurological patient, hyperkalaemia can occur after the administration of succinylcholine to patients who have severe burns, peripheral neuropathy or spinal cord injury all associated with significant denervation of muscle.

Hypokalaemia

Hypokalaemia may be due to excessive hyperventilation, stress-induced sympathetic stimulation, or diuretic therapy, and is included in the differential diagnosis of muscle weakness. Hypokalaemia may also be associated with cardiac conduction and rhythm abnormalities which may be potentiated by the administration of digoxin. Treatment requires an evaluation of the chronicity of hypokalaemia. Chronic hypokalemia should be reversed slowly using the enteral route if possible. Intravenous therapy is frequently required for patients at risk of cardiovascular complications.

Calcium

Calcium is essential for nerve and muscle excitability and contractility, and derangements in calcium concentrations are rare in the neurologic intensive care unit. A more common finding of hypocalcemia in the intensive care patient occurs with extensive blood transfusions.

Magnesium

Magnesium is another important ion for contractility of the heart and at the neuromuscular junction. The central nervous system effects are less prominent. Patients with impaired renal function are susceptible to hypermagnesaemia as elimination is primarily through the kidney. Hypermagnesaemia can be treated with administration of calcium in the acute phase. Fluid loading and diuresis is used in patients with competent renal function; however, dialysis may be necessary.

Hypomagnesaemia can occur from malabsorption syndromes including alcoholism and in gastrointestinal disorders involving diarrhoea and vomiting. Patients with hypomagnesaemia present with hyperreflexia, muscle spasm and seizures. Cardiac irritability and an increased risk of digoxin-induced cardiac dysrhythmias may occur. Hypomagnesaemia can be treated by administration of intravenous magnesium sulphate 1–2 g over 30–60 min to reverse the cardiovascular and neurologic side-effects. Magnesium sulphate administration can be monitored at the bedside by evaluating depression in the tendon reflexes.

Phosphate

Neurologically impaired individuals may have inadequate nutrition leading to hypophosphataemia. Re-administration of nutritional supplement to these patients induces severe hypophosphataemia, as part of a refeeding syndrome. Phosphate levels in the blood can drop precipitously causing a variety of central nervous system effects including decreased level of consciousness. Most frequently, however, hypophosphataemia presents with diffuse neuromuscular weakness which may also affect muscles of respiration requiring mechanical ventilation. Phosphate should be repleted in large doses orally during refeeding, and should a severe refeeding syndrome occur, intravenous sodium or potassium phosphate should be administered slowly over 2–4 h.

KEY POINTS

- The importance of monitoring and evaluating electrolyte and water disturbances in neurologic disease cannot be understated.
- Brain injury affects sodium and water homeostasis within the body. Shifts in electrolyte and water can affect brain function and worsen cerebral oedema regardless of the cause.
- Understanding the pathological mechanisms behind these abnormal concentrations requires an understanding of the complex interaction of neuroendocrine hormones controlling water and sodium balance.
- The initial evaluation of these syndromes is made easier by first evaluating intravascular volume (Fig. 42.2).
- While neurointensive care patients can experience a variety of electrolyte abnormalities beyond sodium and water, these other electrolyte abnormalities are seen at a frequency similar to the general ICU patient population.

	Diabetes Insipidus	SIADH	Salt Wasting
Serum Sodium	↑ or ↔	↓	↓
Urine Sodium	↔	↔	↑
Urine Osmolality	↓	↑	↔ or ↓
Vascular Volume	↓ or ↔	↔ or ↑	↓
Body Weight	↓	↔ or ↑	↓
Blood Pressure	↓ or ↔	↔ or ↑	↔
CVP	↓	↔	↓

Figure 42.2 Common clinical syndromes in the neurointensive care unit

FURTHER READING

Andrews B 1994 Fluid and electrolyte disorders in neurointensive care. *Neurosurg Clin N Am* W B Saunders, Philadelphia, pp. 707–724.

Bhardwaj A, Ulatowski JA 1999 Cerebral edema: hypertonic saline solutions. *Curr Treatment Options Neurol*. 1: 179–199.

Diringer M 1995 Neuroendocrine regulation of sodium and volume following subarachnoid hemorrhage. *Clin Neuropharmacol*. 18(2): 114–126.

Moses AM, Blumenthal SA, Streeten DH 1985 Acid-base and electrolyte disorders associated with endocrine disease: pituitary and thyroid: In: Arief A, De Fronzo RA (eds) Fluid, electrolyte and acid-base disorders. Churchill Livingstone. New York pp. 851–892.

43

FLUID MANAGEMENT

J. Monteiro

INTRODUCTION

The goal of initial fluid therapy in a patient with neurologic injury is to restore intravascular volume, optimise haemodynamic parameters and maintain tissue perfusion, integrity and function. The selection of fluids for resuscitation in patients who have decreased intracranial compliance requires an understanding of the relationship between intravenous fluids, brain water and ICP.

PATHOPHYSIOLOGY

Cerebral autoregulation and the *BBB* are two protective mechanisms that may be affected in a patient with neurologic injury.

The influence of **Cerebral autoregulation** on cerebral blood flow and oxygen delivery is discussed in Chapter 5.

The **BBB** is composed of brain endothelial cells with tight junctions creating an effective pore size of 0.7–0.9 nm. These tight junctions are permeable only to water, hence an osmotic gradient is produced by small molecules and ions. Thus even small increases in the concentrations of plasma electrolytes can exert a large osmotic pressure gradient across the BBB and redistribute water to the intravascular space. Normally changes in oncotic pressure do not significantly influence the osmotic pressures in the brain. However, if the BBB is damaged it becomes permeable to a variety of molecules and hydrostatic pressure then becomes important in determining brain water content.

PHARMACOLOGY

The osmotic properties of intravenous fluids are important in determining their efficacy and safety for use in the presence of neurologic injury. (Table 43.1).

Table 43.1 Osmolality of replacement fluids

Fluid	Osmolality mosm/l
7.5% NaCl	2400
25% Mannitol	1100
0.9% NaCl	308
6% Hetastarch	310
Plasma	285
Lactated ringers	250–260
5% Dextrose	252

ISOTONIC FLUIDS

Normal saline is isotonic with an osmolarity of 308 mosm/l and is a useful crystalloid for volume expansion. The overall efficacy of normal saline as a resuscitative fluid is well established but it requires four times the volume of blood lost to restore haemodynamic parameters. Since it is isotonic it has a negligible effect on brain water and in large quantities it may cause a brief rise in brain volume secondary to the increase in intravascular volume.

Gelatins are modified collagen derivatives with a molecular weight of approximately 35,000 Da. Modified fluid gelatin (Gelofusine®) is a 4% solution in normal saline whereas urea-bridged gelatin is a 3.5% solution in normal saline (Haemaccel®). Both are effective plasma volume expanders with an intravascular half-life of 2–3 hours. The low molecular weight leads to rapid renal elimination. The most significant toxicity is anaphylactoid reactions. Depression of fibrinonectin levels and dilutional coagulopathy is possible with the administration of large volumes but no independent defect in haemostasis is noted.

Hydroxyethyl starch solutions contain particles of various molecular weights and degrees of hydroxyethyl substitution, resulting in extremely heterogenous mixtures. Clinically it is available as a 6% solution in normal saline. It has an average molecular weight of 69,000 Da. The oncotic pressure of the solution is 30 mmHg and it has an osmolarity of 310 mosm/l. The kinetics of the entire infusion are complex, with 90% of the infusion eliminated in 42 days although the effective plasma volume expander effects last for 3–24 hours. Tissues such as the liver, spleen and the reticuloendothelial system retain molecules which do not appear to be detrimental to organ function. The product insert recommends a dose limit of 1500 ml or 20 ml/kg/day. However, in cerebrovascular disease the dose should be restricted to 500 ml because of the risk of intracranial bleeding.

HYPERTONIC FLUIDS

Hypertonic Saline

Saline (3%, 10% and 23.4%) has been shown to be effective in reducing ICP in patients with resistant intracranial hypertension by decreasing brain water content by osmosis. It also increases cardiac output, decreases peripheral and cerebrovascular resistance thereby decreasing intracranial pressure. Its use is economical and free from infectious risk, although it is associated with increases in plasma osmolarity, sodium and chloride levels and hypokalemia. Cerebral dehydration and central pontine myelinosis due to rapid changes in serum sodium levels are possible. Recommendations for the use of hypertonic saline are close monitoring of serum sodium levels (less than 160 meq/l) and serum osmolarity (less than 350 mosm/l).

HYPOTONIC FLUIDS

Dextrose (5%) was traditionally given perioperatively in an effort to prevent hypoglycaemia and to limit protein catabolism. However, surgical and traumatic stress normally stimulates gluconeogenesis. Only infants and patients receiving insulin or drugs that interfere with glucose synthesis are at a significant risk of hypoglycaemia. Glucose infusions are known to produce hyperglycaemia in neurosurgical patients even in moderate doses. In humans, hyperglycaemia is associated with worse outcomes in both ischaemic and traumatic brain injury. The dextrose in water is quickly metabolised, leaving free water. These hypotonic solutions thus increase brain water due to the osmotic gradient.

FLUID MANAGEMENT

FLUID RESUSCITATION

Neurosurgical procedures and isolated HI are associated with minimal losses of extracellular fluid, although associated injuries may necessitate aggressive fluid replacement. Surgical and traumatic losses in patients at risk for intracranial hypertension can be replaced with 0.9% saline or colloid. Substantial or chronic loss of gastrointestinal fluids requires replacement of other electrolytes (i.e. potassium, magnesium, phosphate). Replacement of fluid losses also must compensate for sequestration of interstitial fluid that accompanies trauma, haemorrhage and tissue manipulation. Based on estimates of fluid sequestration associated with extensive tissue manipulation, simple guidelines have been developed for replacement of third space losses. The simplest formula provides, in addition to maintenance fluids and replacement of estimated blood loss, 4 ml/kg/h for procedures involving minimal trauma, 6 ml/kg/h for those involving moderate trauma and 8–15 ml/kg/h for those involving severe trauma.

COMMONLY ENCOUNTERED FLUID ABNORMALITIES IN NEUROINTENSIVE CARE

Cerebral Salt Wasting Syndrome

This is caused by the release of atrial natriuretic factor (ANF) in response to SAH or areas of cerebral injury.

ANF increases renal sodium excretion thereby causing a decrease in plasma volume. Cerebral salt wasting syndrome is characterised by hyponatremia, hypovolemia, and a urine sodium > 50 mmol/l. The management involves rapid restoration of the blood volume and the recommended fluid for resuscitation is 0.9% saline.

SIADH

The syndrome of inappropriate antidiuretic hormone secretion (SIADH) often is associated with ectopic neoplastic ADH secretion or excessive hypothalamic-pituitary release of ADH secondary to neurologic pathologic states, pain, surgery or neuroendocrine abnormalities. It is characterised by a urinary sodium of > 20 mmol/l, hyponatremia, hypervolemia and hyposmolarity. It is managed by free water restriction sufficient to reduce total body water by 0.5–1.0 l/day. The resultant reduction in glomerular filtration rate enhances proximal tubular reabsorption of salt and water and stimulates aldosterone secretion. Demeclocycline (a tetracycline) or lithium antagonise the renal actions of ADH in refractory cases of SIADH. Neurological symptoms with profound hyponatremia (serum Na^+ < 115–120 meq/l) requires aggressive therapy. Three per cent saline is indicated in patients who have seizures or who develop signs of water intoxication. Three per cent saline at a rate of 1–2 ml/kg/h to increase serum Na^+ by 1–2 meq/l/h can be used and should be monitored every 1–2 hours to avoid over-correction.

Diabetes Insipidus

This is common following pituitary and hypothalamic lesions and can also occur with other cerebral pathology such as head trauma and intracranial surgery. It is characterised by polyuria, dehydration, hypernatremia, a low urinary sodium and a low urine specific gravity. It is managed according to whether its aetiology is central or nephrogenic. Central diabetes insipidus requires exogenous replacement of ADH with either desmopressin (DDAVP) or aqueous vasopressin. DDAVP may be given subcutaneously in a dose of 1–4 μg every 12–24 hours or intra-nasally in a dose five times larger. Incomplete ADH deficits (partial diabetes insipidus) are effectively managed with chlorpropamide 250–750 mg/day, clofibrate, 250–500 mg/6–8 hours or carbamazepine, 400–1000 mg/day. Nephrogenic diabetes insipidus is managed by restricting sodium and water intake and hydrochlorothiazide, 50–100 mg/day.

KEY POINTS

- Early detection and correction of fluid abnormalities helps in minimising cerebral oedema.
- Osmotic gradients occur across the BBB.
- Isotonic solutions (crystalloid and colloids) are good resuscitation fluids. A greater volume of crystalloid is required due to redistribution.
- Hypertonic saline is useful in reducing cerebral oedema and ICP after brain injury.
- Avoid glucose containing fluids except in hypoglycaemia.
- Do not fluid restrict unless the patient is fluid overloaded or has SIADH.

FURTHER READING

Sutin KM, Ruskin KJ, Kaufman BS. Intravenous fluid therapy in neurologic injury. Crit Care Clin 1992; 8 (2): 367–408

Tommassino C, Moore S, Todd MM. Cerebral effects of isovolemic hemodilution with crystalloid or colloid solutions. Crit Care Med 1988; 16: 862

Damon L, Adams M, Sticker RB. Intracranial bleeding during treatment with hyroxyethyl starch. N England J Med 1987; 317: 964

Longstreth WT, Inui TS. High blood glucose level on hospital admission and poor neurological recovery after cardiac arrest. Ann Neurol 1984; 15: 59–63

Campbell IT, Baxter JN, et al. IV fluids during surgery. Br J Anaes 1990; 65: 726

44

SEDATION

J. Monteiro

INTRODUCTION

Sedation in neurointensive care is used to minimise cerebral metabolic demands following injury to balance the effects of large amounts of circulating catecholamines, and to help control intracranial hypertension. The actual level of sedation required varies enormously. Patients recovering from uneventful craniotomy require less sedation and analgesia than those with multiple trauma and refractory intracranial hypertension. Indications for sedation are shown in Table 44.1.

PHARMACOLOGY

The pharmacodynamic effects of sedative medications are influenced by the complexity of critical illness. Combinations of analgesic, sedating and tranquillising agents help to individualise patient-specific therapy. Short-acting drugs are commonly used either intermittently or more usually, as a continuous infusion (Table 44.2).

ANALGESICS (see Chapter 10)

Morphine is sometimes used as the sole agent or in combination with neuromuscular blocking drugs, particularly in the USA. Its analgesic properties last for 2–4 hours as a bolus and there is an associated sedative effect. It is metabolised to morphine-6-glucuronide, an active compound, which accumulates in renal failure. Shorter-acting agents (e.g. fentanyl, alfentanil) should be used in renal dysfunction. Fentanyl has no active metabolites but significant amounts may accumulate with prolonged administration as elimination half-life depends on the duration of continuous infusion. The residual sedative and respiratory depressant effects of long-term fentanyl infusions may also last well beyond any analgesic effects. Remifentanil may be useful but is expensive and unlicensed for intensive care use.

Table 44.1 Indications for sedation in neurointensive care

- Control intracranial pressure
- Decrease cerebral metabolism
- Facilitate mechanical ventilation
- Provide amnesia during paralysis with muscle relaxants
- Treat status epilepticus
- Relieve anxiety and fear; facilitate sleep
- Provide haemodynamic stability

SEDATIVES AND ANXIOLYTICS

Midazolam is a water-soluble, non-analgesic benzodiazepine giving peak sedation within 5–10 minutes. The duration of sedative effect ranges from 3 to 120 minutes and the elimination half-life is 2–4 hours. The active metabolite 1-hydroxymidazolam is 60–80% as potent as the parent drug and undergoes renal elimination with a half-life of 1 hour. Reports of prolonged sedation with midazolam are related to the pharmacokinetics, which are markedly altered in critically ill patients.

Propofol shows a linear relationship between infusion rate and steady-state blood concentration allowing easy titration in the intensive care setting. It can be safely used in patients with altered intracranial compliance. Infusion at a rate of 2–4 mg/kg/h in severe HI provides satisfactory sedation without changes in CPP. Serum lipid levels may increase following prolonged infusion due to the formulation in oil emulsion and altered lipid clearance in critical illness. Serum triglyceride levels should be monitored and parenteral nutrition supplements adjusted accordingly. Care must be taken with induced hypothermia, which further reduces lipase activity and hepatic clearance.

Propofol is usually preferred to midazolam if a short period of sedation is anticipated or fast reversal of sedation is planned (e.g. neurological reassessment, weaning from ventilation, performance of brainstem death criteria).

Table 44.2 Drug dosages for intravenous sedation

	Bolus	Infusion
Morphine	0.1–0.2 mg/kg	0.05–0.07 mg/kg/h
Fentanyl	2–5 µg/kg	1–10 µg/kg/h
Alfentanil	10–25 µg/kg	10–50 µg/kg/h
Midazolam	0.2–1 mg/kg	20–200 µg/kg/h
Propofol	1–2 mg/kg	2–10 mg/kg/h

MUSCLE RELAXANTS

Neuromuscular blocking drugs are frequently used to synchronise ventilation, manipulate $PaCO_2$ and minimise increases in ICP. Atracurium is commonly given, tolerated well haemodynamically and has few drug interactions. Laudanosine, a metabolite produced by Hoffman elimination is not a clinical problem in humans. Pancuronium boluses are occasionally used, guided by a peripheral nerve stimulator. Generally, the steroid-based agents are best avoided in critical illness.

MONITORING LEVEL OF SEDATION

Sedation scales have been described that are easy to use but they cannot discriminate between subtle changes in the level of sedation or distinguish different levels from abnormal mental states. No satisfactory objective clinical measure of sedation exists and therapy is usually guided by intermittent clinical assessment. Use of sedation scales is precluded when neuromuscular blocking agents are administered.

Non-pharmacological methods should also be considered to provide relief from the stressful intensive care environment. Efforts to reduce noise and lighting, good communication and education, restoration of privacy, a flexible visiting policy, and reinstitution of patient control may provide relief from anxiety. Treatable causes of agitation and confusion such as hypoxia, hypercarbia, hypoglycaemia, electrolyte disorders, drug or alcohol withdrawal, pain, sleep deprivation, organic psychosis, meningitis or other systemic infections, and ischaemic or thrombotic cerebrovascular events should be investigated before sedation is initiated or increased to treat anxiety or combativeness.

KEY POINTS

- Sedation aims to optimise cerebral perfusion and oxygenation.
- Combinations of sedatives and analgesics are commonly used.
- Neuromuscular paralysis is frequently used if ICP is elevated.
- Causes of agitation need to be identified and treated prior to sedation.
- No satisfactory objective clinical measure of sedation exists.

FURTHER READING

Butterworth JB, DeWitt DS. Severe head trauma: pathophysiology and management. Crit Care Clin 1989; 5: 807

Aitkenhead AR, Pepperman ML, Willatts SM, et al. Comparison of propofol and midazolam for sedation in critically ill patients. Lancet 1989; 2: 704

Farling PA, Johnston JR, Coppel DL. Propofol infusion for sedation of patients with head injury in intensive care: a preliminary report. Anaesthesiology 1989; 44: 222

Hansen-Flaschen J, Cowan J, Polomano R. Beyond the Ramsay scale: need for a validated measure of sedating drug efficiency in the intensive care unit. Crit Care Med 1994; 22: 732

Park GR, Sladen RN (eds). Sedation and analgesia in the critically ill. Oxford: Blackwell Science, 1995

Wheeler A. Sedation, analgesia and paralysis in the intensive care unit. Chest 1993; 104: 566–577

45

COAGULATION DISORDERS

P. Doyle

INTRODUCTION

Haemostasis is a continual dynamic equilibrium between the clotting cascade and the fibrinolytic system, the vascular endothelium and adequately functioning platelets. It is imperative to correct any coagulation abnormalities early to minimise mass effects of intracranial bleeding and haematoma formation.

PATHOPHYSIOLOGY

A number of transient but normal physiological responses may occur during elective neurosurgery (Table 45.1).

Table 45.1 Normal haemostatic response to brain injury	
Haemostatic Response	Mechanisms (via increased levels of:)
Activation of coagulation	Thrombin; antithrombin
Activation of fibrinolysis	Plasmin-antiplasmin; d-Dimers
Activation of platelets	β-thromboglobulin; platelet-factor-4
Acute phase response	Fibrinogen; α2-antiplasmin activity

The following events may accompany and influence the above processes including thrombocytopaenia, platelet dysfunction, haemodilution, ongoing haemorrhage, hypocalcaemia, acidosis and hypothermia.

Following brain injury, the magnitude of intravascular coagulation is proportional to the amount of intracranial blood and injured brain tissue. The following hypotheses may play a role:

1. Damaged brain tissue contains large amounts of tissue thromboplastin, which enters the circulation and activates the coagulation pathway.
2. Dissolving clot in the subarachnoid space also enters the circulation with CSF and activates the coagulation system.
3. Rapid rises in intracranial pressure or severe meningeal stimulation may induce systemic activation of haemostatic systems through unknown neurogenic and/or humoral mechanisms.

Fibrinolytic activity matches fibrin generation and clot is rapidly cleared, making consumption of clotting factors rather than microthrombosis the primary pathologic event.

MANAGEMENT

Prothrombin time, activated partial thromboplastin time, platelet count, fibrinogen and D-dimer levels test routine coagulation disorders. If time allows, a number of further tests may be employed to specifically look for abnormal bleeding profiles including specific clotting assays (e.g. clotting factor levels, antithrombin, plasminogen, protein C and complexes of thrombin-antithrombin and plasmin-antiplasmin).

Pre-existing coagulation defects, haemorrhage from other injuries and hypothermia need urgent attention. There is a significant prolongation in clotting time for every degree decrease in temperature. Clinical bleeding may be observed in the hypothermic patient in the presence of normal laboratory values performed at 37°C – an important point to remember when induced hypothermia is used as a neuroprotective strategy.

More extensive brain injury is associated with greater disruption of the coagulation/fibrinolytic system. Checks on clotting status should be performed early and regularly. Abnormalities should be corrected with transfusions of fresh frozen plasma, cryoprecipitate and platelets as indicated. If a screen for DIC has elevated D-dimer levels and minimal other abnormalities, the tests should be repeated within two hours to ascertain progress and the advice of a haematologist sought.

KEY POINTS

- Brain tissue levels of thromboplastin are high and are potent stimulants of the coagulation cascade, fibrinolytic system and platelet activation.
- Severe brain injury and intracranial haemorrhage activates these pathways more than lesser injuries.
- Coagulopathy is a risk factor for adverse outcome in brain injured patients.
- Perform early assessment and correction of clotting abnormalities.

RECOMMENDED READING

Fujii Y, Takeuchi S et al. 1995 Hemostasis in spontaneous subarachnoid hemorrhage. *Neurosurgery* 37(2), 226–234.

Hulke F, Mullins RJ, Frank EH. 1996 Blunt brain injury activates the coagulation process. *Archives of Surgery* 131: 923–928.

Levine SR, Tietjen GE, Dafer R, Feldman E. 1999 Hematologic abnormalities and stroke. In: Ginsberg MD, Bogousalavsky J, eds. *Cerebrovascular Disease. Pathophysiology, diagnosis and management*. Mass. USA: Blackwell Science, pp. 1698–1726.

Rohrer MJ, Natale AM. 1992 Effect of hypothermia on the coagulation cascade. *Critical Care Medicine* 20, 1402-1405.

46

STATUS EPILEPTICUS

N. Hirsch

DEFINITION AND INCIDENCE

Generalised convulsive status epilepticus (GCSE), the most common form of status epilepticus, may be defined as a condition in which continuous or rapidly repeating tonic-clonic seizures persist for 30 minutes or more. Its incidence is approximately 25 per 100,000 of the population and it is estimated that 9–14,000 cases occur annually in the UK. In about one-third of cases, GCSE is the first presentation of epilepsy.

Overall mortality of adult GCSE is approximately 20%.

AETIOLOGY

The aetiology of adult GCSE may be conveniently divided into acute and chronic processes (see Table 46.1).

CLINICAL FEATURES

During the initial stages of GCSE, the diagnosis is apparent, with tonic and clonic movements of the limbs in an unresponsive, often incontinent patient. However, in the later stages the movements often become subtle with only minor twitching of the face, eyelids, hands or feet. It is vital to recognise this stage as treatment must be rapid to avoid permanent cerebral damage (see below).

PATHOPHYSIOLOGY

The physiological derangement that occurs in GCSE is often divided into two phases, the second occurring after approximately 30 minutes of seizure activity.

During *Phase 1*, the increased cerebral metabolic demand is satisfied by an increase in CBF and an increase in autonomic activity resulting in increased arterial blood pressure, increased blood glucose levels, sweating, hyperpyrexia and salivation.

Phase 2 is characterised by a failure of cerebral autoregulation, a rise in ICP and hypotension resulting in decreased cerebral perfusion. Hypoxaemia occurs due to decreased central respiratory drive, pulmonary hypertension and oedema, cardiac failure and the increased oxygen demand. At this stage, oxygen delivery cannot keep pace with demand, and electromechanical dissociation may occur, in which although electrical cerebral seizure activity continues, its clinical manifestations may be restricted to minor twitching. The longer the attack lasts the less responsive it becomes to therapy and the greater the chance of permanent brain damage, especially to limbic structures such as the hippocampus. This damage is further compounded by the systemic complications described above.

Other complications include acute tubular necrosis, rhabdomyolysis, hypoglycaemia, lactic acidosis, multi-organ failure and disseminated intravascular coagulation.

MANAGEMENT

Morbidity and mortality of GCSE is directly related to the duration of the seizures and therefore management should be rapid and effective. It is conveniently divided into general management and drug therapy.

GENERAL MANAGEMENT

Assessment of cardiopulmonary function should be carried out immediately and oxygen administered. Tracheal intubation is necessary if the airway is compromised or hypoxaemia continues despite administration of oxygen by mask. If intubation is necessary, a short-acting neuromuscular blocking agent (e.g. atracurium) should be used so that the ability to detect clinical seizures is rapidly regained. Intravenous access should be established and a blood glucose assay performed. *50 ml of 50% glucose* should

---

Table 46.1 Aetiology of generalised convulsive status epilepticus in adults

Acute processes	Chronic processes
• Electrolyte imbalance (e.g. Na^+, Ca^{++} etc.) • Renal failure • Sepsis syndrome • Head injury • Cerebrovascular accident • Drug toxicity (e.g. cocaine, alcohol abuse) • CNS infection – encephalitis, meningitis • Hypoxic brain injury	• Pre-existing epilepsy • Poor compliance – low anticonvulsant drug levels • Chronic alcoholism • Cerebral tumours or other space occupying lesions

be given if this is low. Any suggestion of malnutrition or chronic alcoholism should be treated with *thiamine (100 mg)* to avoid precipitating Wernicke's encephalopathy.

Following resuscitation, *regular monitoring* of cardiorespiratory function, neurological observations and temperature should be instituted. Anticonvulsant therapy (see below) should be commenced.

Acidosis is often profound in patients with GCSE but usually corrects itself following resuscitation. However, intravenous bicarbonate may be necessary. *Hyperthermia* reflects increased muscle activity and may worsen neuronal damage; passive cooling and rectal paracetamol may be used if the increased temperature persists.

Once emergency treatment has been carried out, a detailed *history* (usually from relatives) and *examination* is performed and this often gives a clue to the aetiology (e.g. previous epilepsy, co-existing medical condition, drug abuse etc.). *Haematological and biochemical studies* should be performed as well as *anticonvulsant drug levels* and a *toxicology screen* if indicated.

Other systemic complications of GCSE described above should be treated in the standard manner.

DRUG THERAPY (see Table 46.2)

GCSE is often heralded by an increase in the intensity or frequency of seizures (the so-called *premonitory stage*). Treatment at this stage may abort evolution into true status. The drugs of choice at this stage are *diazepam, midazolam* or *paraldehyde*.

Early GCSE (within first 30 minutes) is best treated with *diazepam* or *lorazepam*. Repeated doses of diazepam result in a decreased volume of distribution and clearance leading to accumulation and cardiorespiratory depression. Only two doses should be used before lorazepam is given.

If seizures continue despite this therapy, the stage of *established status* has been reached. *Phenytoin* and/or *phenobarbitone* are the drugs of choice at this stage. They must be given in appropriate doses, underdosing being a major factor in failure to control status. More recently *fosphenytoin*, a water-soluble prodrug of phenytoin has been introduced and appears to have a lower incidence of hypotension than its parent drug.

If seizures persist despite therapeutic levels of phenytoin and phenobarbitone, the stage of *refractory status* has been reached. At this stage, patients require transfer to a specialist neurointensive care unit where continuous EEG can be provided. Refractory status requires anaesthesia; traditionally this has been provided by *thiopentone* or *pentobarbitone* but the saturable kinetics of the barbiturates make regular clinical assessment difficult. *Propofol* is emerging as the drug of choice in these patients.

KEY POINTS

- Overall mortality and morbidity is high and directly related to duration of seizures.
- Neurological and systemic complications may occur.
- Cardiorespiratory support is the first step in management of this condition.
- Benzodiazepines may initially help prevent evolution of established *status*.
- Therapeutic doses of phenytoin or phenobarbitone should be given in established *status*.

Table 46.2 Suggested drug treatment of status epilepticus	
	Dosage
Premonitory stage:	
Diazepam	10–20 mg i.v. or rectally repeated once after 15 minutes if necessary
Midazolam	5–10 mg i.m. or rectally repeated once after 15 minutes if necessary
Paraldehyde	10–20 ml 50% rectally or i.v. repeated once after 15–30 minutes if necessary
Early status:	
Lorazepam	0.07 mg/kg i.v.
Established status:	
Phenytoin	15–18 mg/kg i.v. at rate < 50 mg/min
Phenobarbitone	10–15 mg/kg i.v. at rate < 100 mg/min
Refractory status:	
Thiopentone	250 mg bolus then 2–5 mg/kg/h
Propofol	2 mg/kg bolus then 5–10 mg/kg/h

- *Refractory status* should be treated with anaesthetic agents with EEG monitoring in a neurointensive care unit.

FURTHER READING

Lowenstein DH, Alldredge BK. Status epilepticus. N Engl J Med 1998; 338: 970–976

Shorvon S. Status epilepticus: its clinical features and treatment in children and adults. Cambridge: Cambridge University Press, 1994

Walker MC, Howard RS, Smith SJ, Miller DH, Shorvon SD, Hirsch NP. Diagnosis and treatment of status epilepticus on a neurological intensive care unit. Quart J Med 1996; 89: 913–920

47

GUILLAIN–BARRÉ SYNDROME

N. Hirsch

INTRODUCTION

Guillain–Barré syndrome (GBS), is an acute inflammatory neuropathy characterised by a progressive neuropathic weakness and areflexia and is the commonest cause of neuromuscular paralysis seen in the Western world. Approximately one-third of patients with GBS will develop respiratory failure which may be protracted, and therefore patients may occupy intensive care beds for considerable periods.

The incidence of GBS lies between 1–2 per 100,000 of the population. A history of a preceding infection, usually of the upper respiratory or gastrointestinal tract, is found in at least 75% of cases. Bacterial and viral triggering agents that have been implicated include *Campylobacter jejuni*, *Mycoplasma pneumoniae*, *Epstein–Barr virus*, *human immunodeficiency virus* and *cytomegalovirus*. The use of specific vaccinations (e.g. swine flu vaccine and older preparations of rabies vaccine) has also been associated with outbreaks of GBS.

PATHOPHYSIOLOGY

The association of GBS with preceding infection suggests an immune basis for the inflammatory demyelination of peripheral nerves. Animal models of the condition suggest a cell-mediated process, but the presence of a large variety of complement-fixing antibodies found in patients with GBS correlates with the degree of demyelination seen; furthermore, recovery is associated with a fall in antibody levels.

More recently, an association between an anti-ganglioside antibody (GM1) and *C. jejuni* infection suggests that antibodies raised to this infecting agent may cross-react with the ganglioside of host neural tissue.

CLINICAL FEATURES AND DIAGNOSIS

GBS is an acute neuropathic weakness of more than one limb, areflexia and a duration of progression of fewer than 4 weeks. By convention, disease progressing for longer periods is termed *chronic inflammatory demyelinating polyneuropathy*.

Criteria necessary for diagnosis may be divided into essential and supportive criteria (Table 47.1). Differential diagnosis is found in Table 47.2.

Neurological features

GBS usually presents with pain (especially of the back and sides), mild sensory symptoms (e.g. glove and stocking parathesiae) and relatively symmetrical weakness. The latter often starts in the legs before affecting the arms (hence 'ascending polyneuropathy') and is more pronounced proximally. Cranial nerves (especially the facial nerve and bulbar nerves) are frequently affected.

The Miller–Fisher syndrome has been classified as a variant of GBS and is characterised by ataxia, ophthalmoplegia and areflexia. It is usually associated with anti GQ1b antibodies and often has little in the way of limb weakness.

Respiratory features

Respiratory muscle weakness requiring positive pressure ventilation occurs in 25–30% of patients. Bulbar weakness predisposing to pulmonary aspiration occurs in a similar proportion and may require tracheal intubation for airway protection.

Autonomic dysfunction

Sinus tachycardia is the most common manifestation of autonomic dysfunction and occurs in 75% of

---

Table 47.1 Diagnostic criteria for Guillain–Barré syndrome

Essential criteria	Supportive criteria
• Progressive weakness of more than one limb due to neuropathy • Areflexia • Duration of progression less than four weeks	*Clinical features* • Weakness usually progressive • Sensory signs mild • Cranial nerve involvement common • Autonomic dysfunction common *Laboratory features* • CSF – total protein increased after first week (in 80%) • White cell count normal (in 90%) • EMG – nerve conduction slowed suggesting demyelination

Table 47.2 Differential diagnosis of Guillain–Barré syndrome
• Acute myasthenia gravis • Botulism • Acute intermittent porphyria • Lead and organophosphate poisoning • Poliomyelitis • Polymyositis • Transverse myelitis • Shellfish poisoning

patients. More dangerous are the bradyarrhythmias that may occur with even trivial vagal stimulation. Other autonomic features include postural hypotension, excessive sweating and urinary retention.

MANAGEMENT

The management of GBS consists of supportive treatment and specific therapy.

Supportive treatment

Good general medical and nursing care are essential in the treatment of GBS. Patients must be carefully monitored during the acute and progressing phases and early tracheal intubation should be performed if vital capacity falls below 15 ml/kg. If bulbar weakness co-exists, intubation should be carried out earlier. Tracheostomy should be performed early if it is obvious that a prolonged period of ventilation will be needed.

Sedation is usually given for the first 24 hours following intubation but is not appropriate after this period.

The cardiovascular system must be monitored carefully and persistent tachycardia and hypertension treated with small doses of a β-blocker (e.g. propranolol 5–15 mg daily). Severe episodes of bradycardia warrant temporary or permanent cardiac pacing.

Enteral feeding should be started as soon as possible; however, ileus is common in the acute stages of GBS and may require the use of prokinetic agents such as metoclopramide. Rarely parenteral nutrition may be needed.

Regular turning of the patient with GBS is essential to help prevent pressure sores; passive physiotherapy and the use of limb splints helps to prevent tendon contractures.

Thromboembolic complications remain a major cause of morbidity and mortality in this group and all patients should be treated with graduated elastic stockings and prophylactic subcutaneous heparin.

Pain occurs in up to 70% of patients with GBS and is often very distressing, especially at night. Although simple analgesics such as aspirin or paracetamol may be effective, patients intermittently require stronger analgesia. Meptazinol is a useful agent, providing good analgesia without the troublesome constipating effects of other opioids. In addition, neurogenic pain is often helped by carbamazepine or amitriptyline.

Specific therapy

Plasma exchange (PE) has been shown in a number of large, well-conducted trials to accelerate recovery. Patients likely to benefit most are those who are exchanged within 1 week of the onset of symptoms and those with rapid deterioration of limb power; no benefit is seen if the exchange is performed after 2 weeks of onset. Typically, the exchange consists of replacing 250 ml/kg body weight of the patient's plasma with 4.5% human albumin solution. Morbidity relates to exacerbation of co-existing infection and infective and thromboembolic complications of the large-bore cannula used.

Intravenous normal immunoglobulin (IvIg) is as effective as PE in speeding up the rate of recovery in GBS. It has now become the treatment of choice for GBS as it does not require the manpower demanded by PE and has a lower complication rate. A recent study has suggested that the combination of IvIg and methylprednisolone may be more effective than IvIg alone.

PROGNOSIS

Mortality of GBS varies between 2 and 13%. Typical mortality for patients requiring respiratory support and nursed in a specialised unit is approximately 5%. In general, 25% of patients will be left with a degree of disability 1 year after the onset of GBS.

KEY POINTS

- Triggering agents may be bacterial or viral.
- The disease causes neurological and other systemic effects.
- As well as supportive therapy, the preferred specific treatment includes intravenous immunoglobulin therapy.

FURTHER READING

Hughes RA. Guillain–Barré syndrome. London: Springer-Verlag, 1990

Ng KKP, Howard RS, Fish D, Hirsch NP, et al. Management and outcome of severe Guillain–Barré syndrome. Quart J Med 1995; 88: 243–250

Winer JB. Guillain-Barré syndrome. In: Miller DH, Raps EC (eds) Critical care neurology. Boston: Butterworth-Heinemann, 1999, 33–49

48

TRACHEOSTOMY

Q. Milner

INTRODUCTION

Tracheostomy is one of the oldest recorded surgical procedures and was practised by the ancient Egyptians. Although the indications for tracheostomy have not changed (see below), the introduction of dilatational percutaneous tracheostomies in the 1980s has seen a rapid expansion in their use. Some 12–15% of ICU patients now undergo tracheostomy. This has an effect on ward care after ICU discharge where fewer than 50% of nurses in a study were found to have confidence in detecting and managing a blocked tracheostomy tube and even fewer had received any formal training in managing patients with a tracheostomy.

INDICATIONS FOR TRACHEOSTOMY

- Prolonged ICU ventilation.
- Prolonged tracheo-bronchial toilet.
- Protection of airway and lungs with depressed consciousness and laryngeal reflexes.
- Acute airway obstruction.
- Integral part of a surgical procedure such as laryngectomy.

ADVANTAGES OF TRACHEOSTOMY

Tracheostomy has been established as the airway of choice where either prolonged mechanical ventilation or airway protection is required in the ICU. Sedation and analgesia are rarely needed once a tracheostomy is in place allowing more rapid and controlled weaning, easier access to airway secretions and a potentially shorter ICU stay.

The ideal timing of tracheostomy in patients with neurological deficit has yet to be established. Patients requiring continued ventilation and/or airway protection after 7–10 days of translaryngeal intubation should be considered for tracheostomy unless successful extubation is considered imminent. Important influences on this decision are the degree of continuing neurological deficit (GCS < 8), the presence of respiratory infection and the nature and amount of secretions.

COMPLICATIONS OF TRACHEOSTOMY

Immediate procedural complications

- Haemorrhage.
- Pneumothorax.
- Malposition of tracheostomy tube in peritracheal tissues.
- Tracheal/laryngeal damage.
- Surgical emphysema.
- Ventilator disconnection.
- Hypoxia.

Delayed complications

- Tracheostomy tube obstruction.
- Infection.
- Erosion into tracheal cartilages, oesophagus or blood vessels.

Late complications

- Post-extubation tracheal stenosis.
- Persistent fistula.
- Tracheomalacia.

PERCUTANEOUS TRACHEOSTOMY

Little interest was shown in percutaneous tracheostomy when described by Sheldon in 1957. However, since the description of a Seldinger wire technique for percutaneous dilatational tracheostomy by Pascale Ciaglia in 1985, it has rapidly gained acceptance and may be considered the technique of choice for many ICU patients.

The nature and incidence of perioperative complications and infection has been found to be similar to or better than those associated with surgical tracheostomy. A number of authors believe that direct visualisation of the procedure by an assistant with a fibreoptic bronchoscope may reduce complications still further. More recently, ultrasound-guided insertion has been described which is useful in patients with landmarks that are difficult to palpate or visualise. Particular care should be taken during tracheostomy to avoid hypoventilation with hypercarbia as well as hypoxia in the patient with neurological injury and non-compliant ICP. The incidence of late tracheal stenosis is difficult to quantify since patients may be asymptomatic with greater than 50% narrowing of the trachea and stridor may not occur until tracheal diameter is less than 5 mm.

Percutaneous dilatational tracheostomy is a bedside procedure that can be carried out on any ICU without the need to transfer patients to the operating theatre. This removes the risks of transferring critically ill patients, frees theatre time and staff and allows tracheostomy to occur more rapidly once the decision has been made. Timpson et al[1] have found a doubling of the incidence of tracheostomy since the introduction of percutaneous techniques in one ICU, coupled with a very large decrease in the number of surgical tracheostomies performed.

DECANNULATION OF TRACHEOSTOMY

The initial cuffed tracheostomy tube should be replaced with an uncuffed and subsequently fenestrated (speaking) tracheostomy tube as a part of weaning prior to decannulation of the tracheostomy. The tracheostomy site rarely needs more than an occlusive dressing.

KEY POINTS

- Tracheostomy is useful for prolonged ICU ventilation and tracheo-bronchial toilet.
- It may hasten the weaning process.
- Tracheostomy can be performed surgically or percutaneously by the bedside.
- Tracheostomy should be considered after 7–10 days of ventilation.

FURTHER READING

Hatfield A, Bodenham A. Portable ultrasonic scanning of the anterior neck before percutaneous dilatational tracheostomy. Anaesthesia 1999; 54: 660–663

Holdgaard HO, Pederson J, Jensen RH, et al. Percutaneous dilational tracheostomy versus conventional surgical tracheostomy. Acta Anaethes Scand 1998; 42: 545–550

Plummer AL, Gracey DR. Consensus conference on artificial airways in patients receiving mechanical ventilation. Chest 1989; 96: 712–713

REFERENCE

1. Timpson TP, Day CJE, Jewkes CF, Manara AR. The impact of percutaneous tracheostomy on intensive care unit practice and training. Anaesthesia 1999; 54: 186–189

49

BRAINSTEM DEATH

Q. Milner

INTRODUCTION

The development of artificial ventilation in the 1950s has enabled cardiopulmonary function to be maintained in apnoeic patients with severe intracranial pathology who would otherwise have died. This has changed our understanding of the nature of death and we now define it as 'the irreversible loss of the capacity for consciousness, combined with the irreversible loss of the capacity to breathe'.

As the brainstem maintains consciousness, the sleep–wake cycle and ventilation, death of the brainstem is equivalent to death of the entire brain. Asystole follows brainstem death without exception and may occur within minutes or rarely up to a few weeks after.

The diagnosis of brainstem death allows humanitarian, ethical and economic management of critical care resources and may allow the optimisation of organs for transplantation.

KEY FEATURES

Brainstem death may only be diagnosed in patients with apnoeic coma resulting from known irreversible intracranial pathology. This is most frequently seen in:

* Severe head injury.
* Intracranial haemorrhage.
* Cerebral oedema with brainstem herniation.
* Hypoxic-ischaemic encephalopathy.

A number of exclusions must be satisfied before the diagnosis of brainstem death may be made including the absence of:

* Depressant drugs which may cause unconsciousness.
* Hypothermia (< 35°C).
* Severe hypotension.
* Gross endocrine, biochemical and metabolic abnormality.
* Abnormal $PaCO_2$.

DIAGNOSTIC TESTS TO CONFIRM BRAINSTEM DEATH

In the UK, two doctors carry out the brainstem death tests according to a strict protocol. One doctor must be a consultant and the other must be qualified for at least 5 years. If organs are to be transplanted, neither doctor may be a member of the transplant team. The tests should be carried out more than 6 hours after the events leading to brainstem death. UK law requires only one set of tests but it is common to repeat the tests

after an interval of at least 30 minutes. The time of death is noted at completion of the first set of tests:

Pupillary Reflexes

Pupillary response to bright light should be absent in both eyes. This tests afferent pathways of the optic nerve (CN II) and efferent pathways of the oculomotor nerve (CN III). Pupil size is irrelevant and normal doses of atropine have no effect on this reflex.

Corneal reflex

Corneal reflexes should be tested with cotton wool in the lateral part of the cornea. (CN V and VII).

Facial sensation and motor responses

Firm pressure on the supra-orbital ridge should elicit no facial responses (CN V and VII). Spinal cord reflexes may persist in brainstem death.

Oculocephalic reflex (Doll's eye movement)

This test should not be carried out in the presence of cervical spine fracture. Rapid lateral movement of the head normally results in eye deviation to the contralateral side, testing brainstem gaze mechanisms. In brainstem death the eyes remain in a fixed position within the orbit.

Caloric testing

This tests vestibular reflexes in CN VIII. Both ears are irrigated with 20–30 ml ice cold water after inspection of the intact drum. Nystagmus to the stimulated side is absent in brainstem death.

Gag and cough reflexes

The gag and cough reflexes are absent in response to a pharyngeal and tracheal stimulus (CN IX and X).

Apnoea testing

Normocapnoea should be achieved and the patient ventilated with 100% oxygen for 3 minutes prior to disconnection from the ventilator. Apnoeic oxygenation is achieved by placing a catheter with oxygen flowing at 4 l/min in the trachea. The patient is inspected for signs of respiration for 10 minutes or until arterial blood gases confirm that the $PaCO_2$ exceeds 6.5 kPa. Significant hypotension and hypoxaemia (SaO_2 < 90%) should be avoided.

Further tests

The above tests are sufficient for the diagnosis of brainstem death in the UK and USA. Some other countries require confirmatory tests such as EEG, transcranial Doppler ultrasonography and angiography, but there is no evidence that these tests contribute to the diagnosis.

CHILDREN

The British Paediatric Association (1991) have stated that for children over the age of 2 months, brainstem death criteria should be the same as for adults.

PERSISTENT VEGETATIVE STATE (PVS)

Patients in PVS have suffered cortical damage and do not meet the basic criteria for brainstem death testing; these two conditions should not be confused.

SUBSEQUENT MANAGEMENT

Organ donation should only be discussed with patient's relatives after the diagnosis of brainstem death has been made. The family should be clear that despite the presence of a beating heart, the patient is dead and ventilation may legally be ceased. If organ donation is planned, the focus of patient care should be redirected to optimising organ function prior to transplantation (see Chapter 64).

KEY POINTS

- An irreversible intracranial event causing apnoea must be identified.
- Patients need to satisfy all brainstem death criteria.
- Brainstem death criteria should be carried out on two occasions by qualified medical staff.
- Time of death is noted after the first set of tests.

FURTHER READING

Department of Health. A Code of Practice for the diagnosis of Brain Stem Death. Health Service Circular, 1998

Jennett B. Brain death. Intens Care Med 1982; 8: 1–3

Milner QJW, Vuylsteke A, Ismail F, Ismail-Zade I, Latimer RD. ICU resuscitation of the multi-organ donor. Br J Intens Care 1997; 2: 49–54

Wijdicks EFM. Determining brain death in adults. Neurology 1995; 45: 1003–1011

50

NUTRITION IN THE NEUROCRITICAL CARE UNIT

Q. Milner

INTRODUCTION

The provision of adequate nutritional support is an essential component of caring for the critically ill patient. During starvation, homeostatic mechanisms are designed to burn fat rather than protein as an energy source until the fat stores are significantly depleted. The catabolic state that occurs in critical illness, however, ensures significant protein loss from early in the illness.

Moderate to severe head injury is characterised by the development of an hypermetabolic and hypercatabolic state. Plasma and urine levels of catecholamines and cortisol are elevated. Hyperglycaemia occurs frequently and is a major cause of ketone production, increasing lactic acid production by the brain and cellular acidosis. The severity and duration of hyperglycaemia following head injury has been shown to correlate with longer term outcome. Efforts to avoid hyperglycaemia are important.

Immune suppression occurs in head-injured patients with a decrease in the T cell lymphocyte CD4/CD8 ratio. The early instigation of effective nutritional support may decrease secondary neurological injury and improve outcome.

ENTERAL NUTRITION

Enteral nutrition is preferred in the critically ill. This can be achieved by either nasal tube feeding or via a percutaneous gastrostomy (PEG) if prolonged feeding is envisaged. Standard enteral feeding regimes aim to provide 1500–2500 kcal in 24 hours with 70 g protein in a volume of 1.5–2 L. More concentrated feeds and low electrolyte feeds are available for patients in renal failure.

Advantages associated with enteral rather than parenteral nutrition include:

1. Maintenance of mucosal integrity and prevention of villous atrophy.
2. Reduced infection rate.
3. Absence of requirement for central venous line.
4. Better maintenance of fluid balance.
5. Reduced cost.

Contraindications to enteral feeding are few, particularly in the patient with isolated intracranial pathology, but include abdominal sepsis, obstruction, acute malabsorption and inflammatory syndromes and enteric fistulae. Only a short segment of small intestine (30 cm) is required for adequate absorption since hypertrophy will occur in response to lumenal nutrients. Neither bowel sounds nor flatus are required for successful enteral feeding.

Enteral feeding should be started if gastric aspirates are less than 400 ml/day and there are no obvious contraindications. Commence with standard enteral feed at 25 ml/h, increasing the rate every 12 hours until 100 ml/h is achieved. Aspirate residual volume and rest for 1 hour in every 6 hours of feeding, and rest continuously for 8 hours overnight.

COMPLICATIONS OF ENTERAL FEEDING

1. Large residual gastric volumes.
2. Regurgitation and aspiration.
3. Diarrhoea.
4. Ulceration of nares.
5. Contamination of feed (rare).

Gastric atony and delayed emptying occur commonly in HI and may make establishing early enteral feeding difficult. Pro-kinetic agents such as metoclopramide or erythromycin are used to promote gastric motility. A nasojejunal tube may be inserted to bypass the pylorus. The passage of nasal feeding tubes should be avoided in patients with facial injuries and basal skull fracture.

Diarrhoea is also common with enteral feeding and may resolve with a different formula of feed. Persistent diarrhoea may represent infection with *Clostridium difficile*, particularly in patients receiving multiple antibiotics. A specimen should always be sent for microbiological culture. Loperamide (2 mg) in each 500 ml feed and after each loose stool is an effective treatment for simple diarrhoea.

TOTAL PARENTERAL NUTRITION (TPN)

Although protein calorie requirements are more easily met by parenteral nutrition, it is a poor substitute for enteral nutrition. Energy requirements are 1500–2500 kcal/day depending on the patient's catabolic state. Excessive calorie intake, particularly as carbohydrate, serves no purpose, increasing oxygen consumption, carbon dioxide production, the respiratory quotient (RQ) and lipogenesis. The calorie:nitrogen ratio for TPN is 150:1.

TPN should provide:

1. Lipid.
2. Carbohydrates.
3. Amino acids.

4. Electrolytes.
5. Trace elements.
6. Vitamins.

Lipids

Lipids are essential for cell wall integrity, prostaglandin synthesis and the action of fat-soluble vitamins, but should provide no more than 33% of the energy requirements. Intralipid, the only current source of lipid available, is an isotonic emulsion of soyabean oil with egg phosphatides and lecithin. The particle size of the emulsion is similar to a chylomicron, and the lipid is handled in a similar manner. The energy yield from fat is 9 cal/g, but the presence of the egg phosphatides increase the calorific value of intralipid to 11 cal/g.

The lipid load should be decreased in the presence of:

• Sedation with propofol.
• Severe jaundice.
• Severe hypoxaemia.
• Thrombocytopaenia.
• Hypothermia.

Carbohydrates

Two-thirds of the energy requirement is provided by carbohydrate in the form of glucose (energy yield = 4 cal/g). An insulin sliding scale will frequently be required to tightly control plasma glucose levels.

Proteins

Protein is usually omitted from calorific calculations. A wide range of amino acids are supplied as the L-isomer in commercial preparations. Protein requirements increase in sepsis and burns and are 12–17 g nitrogen/day (1 g nitrogen = 6.25 g protein).

Electrolytes

Daily electrolyte requirements of sodium, potassium, calcium, phosphate, magnesium and chloride should be met by TPN.

Trace elements

Trace elements essential for homeostasis include zinc, copper, manganese, iron, cobalt, chromium, selenium, molybdenum and iodine.

Vitamins

Commercially prepared vitamin supplements contain most water-soluble and fat-soluble vitamins (A, D and E) with the exception of folic acid, vitamin B_{12} and vitamin K (fat-soluble).

Increasingly, hospital pharmacies are supplying pre-mixed 'big bag' TPN containing the complete 24-hour nutritional requirements.

KEY POINTS

• HI is associated with the development of an hypermetabolic and hypercatabolic state with immunosuppression.
• Hyperglycaemia worsens brain acidosis and secondary injury and should be avoided.
• Early and effective nutritional support improves longer term outcome after HI.
• Gastric atony and paresis is common following HI.

FURTHER READING

Dark DS, Pingleton SK. Nutrition and nutritional support in critically ill patients. J Intens Care 1993; 8: 16–33

Povlishock J, Bullock MR. Nutritional support of brain-injured patients. J Neurotrauma 1996; 13: 721–729

Robertson CS, Goodman JC, Narayan R, et al. The effects of glucose administration on carbohydrate metabolism after head injury. J Neurosurg 1991; 74: 43–50

51

NURSING ISSUES

S. Rees-Pedlar, S. Walters

INTRODUCTION

The nursing role within a neurointensive care unit requires an in-depth knowledge of factors that contribute to *secondary* brain damage. This is augmented using a range of skills enabling the nurse to effectively assess and monitor the patient and so meet their physical and psychological needs.

NEUROLOGICAL MANAGEMENT

Assessment of neurological status is based primarily on GCS and pupil reaction. Continuous individual management detects early, subtle changes in patient response which may not be reflected in GCS but may reflect deteriorating function (e.g. a higher level of stimulus required to achieve the same response). This one-to-one patient care also facilitates detection of limb and CN deficits, receptive/expressive disorders and impaired muscle tone. The assessment of GCS is limited in sedated patients but small pupil changes (e.g. to ovoid shape) can be significant.

Continuous monitoring of ICP levels and ICP waveform gives information about both early changes in intracranial hypertension and monitor accuracy. Nursing staff are responsible for accurate calibration of monitors after insertion and should ensure the ICP bolt site is kept clean and protected. In the event of uncontrolled rises in ICP, the nurse may be able to promptly identify the cause and take appropriate measures to reduce the pressure (e.g. repositioning).

Accuracy of jugular bulb monitoring relies on regular calibration through jugular venous blood sampling. Recognition of artefact and maintenance of a continuous jugular bulb sensor can be time-consuming. The monitoring catheter is cared for in the same manor as a central line.

RESPIRATORY MANAGEMENT

The degree of respiratory support required varies according to condition. This may range from an assessment of breathing pattern (which may change with rises in ICP) to management of oxygen therapy or the need for positive pressure ventilation. Suctioning is probably the most invasive procedure regularly carried out by nurses in intensive care and so should only be undertaken when indicated by changes in breath sound or blood gas tension. Titration of the effects of chest care on ICP is a major component of nursing care.

Modern ventilator technology allows the critical care practitioner to achieve a desired blood gas tension with a variety of ventilatory modes all of which present different challenges to the nurse. As well as patient safety and comfort during ventilation, maintenance of arterial CO_2 tension is reliant on skilled nursing care.

CARDIOVASCULAR MANAGEMENT

Haemodynamic management and manipulation is important to ensure an adequate CPP. CPP should be continually monitored to determine the parameter causing adverse change (i.e. a fall in MAP or a rise in ICP). It is frequently the nurse who will identify the initiating factor and take appropriate measures to rectify the problem.

Hypertension is often the result of deranged vasomotor control but assessment of other causative factors is essential for correct treatment. Inappropriate sedation levels may cause hypertension in a paralysed, nonsedated patient. Pain and discomfort may also precipitate hypertensive episodes. Simple but important measures such as communicating by speech or touch and comforting may be all that is needed. Particular attention is required with patients who have an unclipped cerebral aneurysm. Untreated hypertension may result in re-bleeding.

Fever has an adverse effect on cerebral metabolism and should be actively managed. Temperature is generally monitored centrally if ICP control is required. Antipyretics and early multiple-site bacterial cultures are employed. Measures to prevent cross-infection should be maintained by all staff. Active cooling may be required to maintain normothermia or induce hypothermia as a means of controlling ICP. Cooling blankets are used to gradually reduce body temperature to desired levels (e.g. 34–35.5°C). This has implications for tissue perfusion, tissue viability and pressure care. Absorption of enteral feed may slow or stop completely.

PAIN AND SEDATION MANAGEMENT

Accurate assessment and appropriate treatment of pain and sedation is ongoing. The use of scoring systems for medical and nursing staff helps give consistent care and analysis of the response to treatment is an important part of the nursing role if treatment is to be successful. As most patients are unable to verbally communicate pain or discomfort, nursing staff will use non-verbal clues such as restlessness or increases in MAP, heart rate and ICP as indications for intervention.

NUTRITION MANAGEMENT

Nutritional requirements in neurointensive care depend on the neurological condition, associated injuries and level of sedation. As with any critically ill patient, it is a primary nursing responsibility to commence and establish enteral nutrition early and research-based feeding guidelines are recommended. Staff should always ascertain correct position of the tube in the stomach before starting feed avoiding the nasal route if base of skull fracture is suspected. Problems with absorption are common due to heavy sedation requirements and gut pro-kinetic agents are frequently required. After feeding is established, a safer and more comfortable long-term feeding tube should be placed. Nursing staff must be extra vigilant to monitor for normoglycaemia and normonatraemia. With continued improvement, eating and drinking should be commenced as appropriate. Problems with swallow or gag reflexes should be referred to a speech therapist for assessment.

ELIMINATION MANAGEMENT

Nursing staff must also be vigilant to monitor hourly and cumulative fluid balances. Salt and water imbalances are common and staff should look for symptoms of common syndromes. Changes in urine volume and concentration can aid in diagnosis and identify the need for laboratory analysis of serum and urine osmolality.

Urinary tract infections are a significant risk to patients who are immobile for many days or weeks, have indwelling catheters and altered immune systems. A major aim of nursing care is to reduce this risk and identify problems early, i.e. good catheter hygiene and regular bacteriological screening.

Gut motility is also impaired through immobility and critical illness. Problems with constipation can continue after the acute phase of illness and can detract from speed of recovery as well as cause distress to the patient. Early bowel assessment and the use of aperients can assist in the management of these problems. Antibiotic use and an impaired immune system leading to diarrhoea are a common problem exacerbated by incontinence. This has implications for skin integrity and patient comfort and dignity and demands skill and attention from the nursing staff.

MOBILITY MANAGEMENT

Nursing skill is required to balance the needs of the patient with clinical condition. Regular assessment is required for the presence of risk factors associated with compromised skin integrity. Frequent position changes are also needed to protect pressure areas as well as aid physiotherapy. Patients should be nursed 'head-up' to prevent decreased venous drainage. Physiotherapy aids early mobilisation of the patient. Mobilising patients out in a chair, using lifting aids as appropriate, assists with physical and psychological care.

HYGIENE MANAGEMENT

Patients are frequently completely dependent on nursing care for hygiene needs. These needs should be balanced against the normal physiological response to fever as frequent washing can affect this response. There is also a need to keep the normal flora of the skin intact. However, the psychological impact of feeling clean and cool together with the therapeutic use of touch and the stimulating smell of familiar products should not be underestimated.

PSYCHOSOCIAL NEEDS

The psychological impact of critical care is well documented but is compounded when the patient also has neurological impairment. Nurses should aim to create an environment that maintains sensory and sleep balance, and involve families in keeping patients in touch with reality. Allowing the patient to reserve some control (when appropriate) and the linking of touch to verbal communication helps to prevent feelings of helplessness and altered body image. Nursing skills are also central to supporting families, partners and friends particularly in the following areas:

- Reducing knowledge deficit.
- Decreasing anxiety and feelings of powerlessness.
- Allowing grief.
- Preventing isolation.

The need for information and hope has always been high in both the critically ill patient and their relative. All members of the multi-disciplinary team have a role in providing this, but it is the nursing staff who are in contact with the patient and family for the longest time periods. They often best gauge patient needs, the family situation and any specific concerns and worries. Good communication between medical and nursing staff is vital if information is to be consistent and family support is to be optimal.

KEY POINTS

The nursing role is multi-faceted and includes:

- Baseline assessment and ongoing patient monitoring.
- Meeting patient needs including sensitive care of psychological, spiritual and social issues.

- Continued support of family and significant others, including education and preparation for future life changes.
- Collaborating with other members of the multi-disciplinary team

FURTHER READING

Gelling L, Prevost AT. A comparison of the perceptions of relatives, nurses and doctors. Care of the Critically Ill. 1999; 15(2): 53–58

Heath DL, Vink R. Secondary mechanisms in traumatic brain injury: a nurse's perspective. Journal of Neuroscience Nursing 1999; 31(2): 97–105

Shah S. Neurological assessment. Nursing Standard 1999. 13(22): 49–54

Section 6

MONITORING

52

INTRACRANIAL PRESSURE

M. Czosnyka

INTRODUCTION

The continuous measurement of ICP is an essential modality in most brain monitoring systems and currently requires an invasive sensor. Attempts to monitor ICP non-invasively (most promisingly with TCD) are still in a phase of technical evaluation.

Measurement of ICP allows us to estimate cerebral perfusion pressure where **CPP = mean arterial blood pressure (ABP) – mean ICP**.

This provides information regarding autoregulation of CBF, compliance of the cerebrospinal system and waveform analysis.

METHODS OF MEASUREMENT

1. *Intraventricular drains*: An external pressure transducer connected to a catheter placed in the ventricular system allowing direct pressure measurement is still considered the 'gold standard' for ICP measurement. Additional advantages include ability for periodic external calibration and CSF drainage. However, insertion of the ventricular catheter may be difficult or impossible in cases of advanced brain swelling and the risk of infection is increased significantly after 3 days of monitoring.
2. *Transducer tipped systems*: Modern ventricular, subdural or intraparenchymal microtransducers reduce infection rates and have excellent metrological properties revealed during bench tests. The intraparenchymal systems may be inserted through an airtight support bolt (e.g. Codman® or Camino® systems) or tunnelled subcutaneously from a burrhole either at the bedside or post craniotomy (Codman® system). With the most common intraparenchymal arrangement however, measured pressure may be localised and not necessarily representative of true ICP (i.e. ventricular CSF pressure). Microtransducers cannot generally be recalibrated after insertion and considerable zero drift may occur during long-term monitoring.
3. *Others*. The least invasive systems available use epidural probes but there is still uncertainty regarding the precise relation between ICP and extradural pressure. Contemporary epidural sensors are now much more reliable than 10 years ago. Lumbar CSF pressure is seldom measured in neurointensive care.

TYPICAL EVENTS AND TRENDS SEEN IN ICP MONITORING

Specific patterns of the ICP waveform can be identified when mean ICP is monitored continuously. Patients with a low and stable ICP (below 20 mmHg) characteristically have no ICP vasogenic waves (Fig. 52.1) with the exception of a phasic response of ICP to rapid variations in arterial blood pressure (ABP). This pattern typically occurs during the initial hours following HJ, before ICP begins to rise.

The most common picture of high but stable ICP (above 20 mmHg) following HI produces vasogenic waves of limited amplitude (Fig. 52.2).

Other examples of ICP waves are shown in Figs 52.3–52.5.

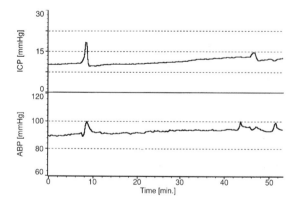

Figure 52.1 Example of ICP and ABP monitoring in patients with low and stable ICP. Characteristically, there are no ICP vasogenic waves (line is very smooth), with exception of a phasic response of ICP to rapid variations in ABP. X-axis is time in minutes

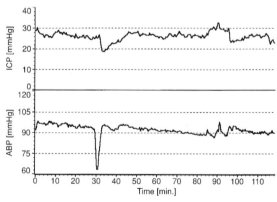

Figure 52.2 Example of a stable but elevated ICP. Vasogenic waves of a limited amplitude are clearly visible along with the response to a rapid (2 min) fall in ABP

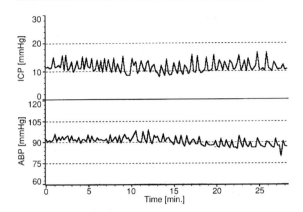

Figure 52.3   Example of regular (30 second) vasogenic ICP B-waves with amplitude 5 mmHg. This pattern is a reflection of the vasocycling often seen in the ABP tracing.

Figure 52.3 shows Vasogenic B waves. Plateau waves are shown in Figure 52.4. Figure 52.5 shows refractory intracranial hypertension (poor prognostic sign).

PULSE WAVEFORM ANALYSIS OF ICP

In order to identify adequate CPPs in individual patients, an analysis of the amplitude of ICP waveforms can be used. The pulse waveform of ICP provides information about the transmission of arterial pulse pressure through the arterial walls to the CSF space. As CPP decreases, the wall tension in reactive brain vessels decreases. This in turn increases transmission of the arterial pulse to ICP. Therefore when cerebral vessels are normally reactive, a decrease in CPP should provoke an increase in the ABP to ICP

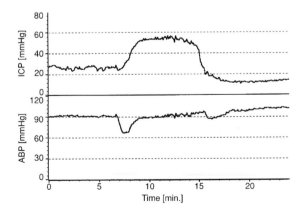

Figure 52.4   Example of a high vasogenic elevation of ICP (plateau wave) caused by a vasodilatation provoked by an initial short-term decrease in ABP

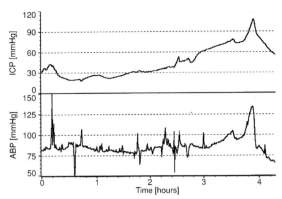

Figure 52.5   Example of a dramatic onset of refractory intracranial hypertension in a patient after severe HI who initially presented with only moderately elevated ICP. After 3 hours of monitoring, ICP increased to above 60 mmHg. The Cushing reflex causing an increase in ABP has been recorded, which ended during the fourth hour with brainstem herniation (demonstrated by a sudden drop in ABP and ICP)

pulse transmission. If this relationship is disturbed the cerebral vessels are no longer pressure-reactive.

A moving linear correlation coefficient between mean ICP and ICP pulse amplitude values termed the RAP index (R = symbol of correlation, A = amplitude, P = pressure) calculated over a 3- to 5-minute time-window is used for continuous detection of the amplitude:pressure relationship. The advantage is that the coefficient has a normalised value from −1 to +1 allowing comparison between patients. The relation of RAP and ICP or CPP in a pooled analysis of patients with HI show a RAP close to +1. This is expected in head-injured patients with a moderately raised ICP (> 15 mmHg) and CPP > 50 mmHg indicating decreased compensatory reserve with preserved cerebrovascular reactivity. A decrease in RAP to 0 or negative values is found with very high ICP and very low CPP and indicates a loss of cerebrovascular reactivity with a risk of brain ischaemia and is also predictive of a poor outcome (Fig. 52.6).

CHANGES IN ICP IN RESPONSE TO VARYING ABP

The correlation between spontaneous waves in ABP and ICP is dependent on the ability of cerebral vessels to autoregulate. With intact autoregulation, a rise in ABP produces vasoconstriction, a decrease in cerebral blood volume, and a fall in ICP. With disturbed autoregulation, changes in ABP are transmitted to the intracranial compartment resulting in a pressure-passive effect.

The correlation coefficient between changes in mean ABP and ICP (termed the PRx index = pressure-reactivity index) is either negative or near to 0 when cerebral vessels are pressure-reactive. A positive correlation coefficient indicates disturbed cerebrovascular pressure-reactivity. This index may fluctuate with time as ICP and CPP varies (Fig. 52.6), but on average it is predictive of outcome.

ICP AND OUTCOME FOLLOWING SEVERE HI

In severe HI, an average ICP above 25 mmHg is associated with a twofold-increased risk of death. In addition, RAP and PRx indices are strong predictors of death, and may be stronger than mean ICP. Good vascular reactivity is an important element of brain homeostasis, enabling the brain to protect itself against uncontrollable rises in intracerebral volume.

KEY POINTS

- Measurement of ICP allows us to estimate CPP.
- The two commonly used methods of measuring ICP are intraventricular catheters with an external transducer or transducer tipped intraparenchymal sensors.
- The PRx reflects autoregulatory reserve of cerebral blood vessels.
- Analysis of the ICP pulse waveform gives useful information regarding adequacy of CPP.

FURTHER READING

Narayan RK, Kishore PR, Becker DP, et al. Intracranial pressure: to monitor or not to monitor? A review of our experience with severe head injury. J Neurosurg 1982; 56(5): 650–659

Czosnyka M, Czosnyka Z, Pickard JD. Laboratory testing of three intracranial pressure microtransducers: technical report. Neurosurgery; 1996, 38: 219–224

Ghajar J. Intracranial pressure monitoring techniques. New Horiz 1995; 3(3): 395–399

Bruder N, N'Zoghe P, Graziani N, Pelissier D, Grisoli F, Francois G. A comparison of extradural and intraparenchymatous intracranial pressures in head injured patients. Intens Care Med 1995; 21(10): 850–852

Portnoy HD, Chopp M, Branch C, Shannon M. Cerebrospinal fluid pulse waveform as an indicator of cerebral autoregulation. J Neurol Neurosurg Psychiatry 1997; 63: 721–731

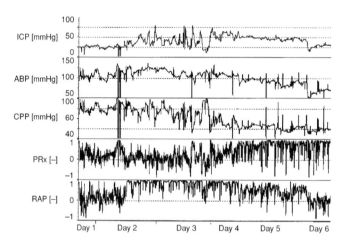

Figure 52.6   Long-term (6 days) monitoring of ICP, ABP, CPP, PRx and correlation coefficient between mean ICP and its pulse amplitude (RAP) in a patient who died following severe HI. Initial ICP was moderately elevated (25 mmHg) with a good compensatory reserve (RAP around 0) and good vascular reactivity (PRx also around 0). On day 2 ICP started to oscillate slowly from 20 to 60 mmHg, RAP increased indicating decrease in cerebrospinal compensatory reserve but PRx remained around 0 indicating good cerebrovascular reactivity. On day 4, PRx increased to positive values (loss of cerebrovascular reactivity) and RAP decreased at a mean ICP of around 50 mmHg (indicating terminal derangement of cerebrovascular responses). Brainstem death was confirmed on day 6

Czosnyka M, Guazzo E, Whitehouse H, et al. Significance of intracranial pressure waveform analysis after head injury. Acta Neurochir (Wien) 1996; 138: 531–542

Czosnyka M, Smielewski P, Kirkpatrick P, Laing RJ, Menon D, Pickard JD. Continuous assessment of the cerebral vasomotor reactivity in head injury. Neurosurgery 1997; 41: 11–19

53

JUGULAR VENOUS OXIMETRY

A.K. Gupta

Jugular venous oximetry ($SjvO_2$) is a method of estimating *global* cerebral oxygenation and metabolism.

INSERTION TECHNIQUE

A catheter is inserted into the internal jugular vein using a Seldinger technique and advanced cephalad beyond the outlet of the common facial vein into the jugular bulb at the base of the skull (Fig. 53.1). Correct placement is confirmed when the catheter tip is level with the mastoid air cells on a lateral neck radiograph.

SITE OF PLACEMENT

It was previously thought that the superior saggital sinus drained into the right IJV and jugular bulb catheters were generally placed on the right to sample the most representative side of the brain. However, more recent data suggest that the venous drainage is less lateralised, and the dominant side of venous drainage can be determined by sequential manual compression of the IJV on each side. The side with the largest rise in ICP is the dominant side and should be cannulated. If the dominant side is not easily detected, the side of the brain with the most pathology is used. In many centres, however, it is still common practice to cannulate the right side, which is usually the dominant IJV. Contraindications and complications are similar to those of an internal jugular CVP line.

METHODS OF MEASUREMENT

Serial samples can be taken to estimate $SjvO_2$, arteriojugular differences in oxygen content ($AJDO_2$),

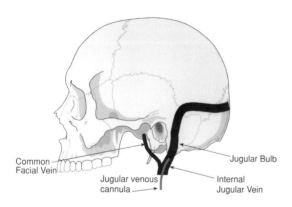

Figure 53.1   Placement of the jugular bulb catheter in the IJV. Note the tip of the sensor should be above the common facial vein

lactate and glucose which is technically easy and cheap. However, this method will only give a 'snapshot' of the state of cerebral oxygenation and metabolism at the time of sampling, and samples may be contaminated by factors such as extracranial venous blood, especially if catheter placement is too low, against the petrosal veins, or if blood sampling is too rapid.

Insertion of fibreoptic catheters enable *continuous monitoring* of $SjvO_2$ with normal values ranging from 60 to 75%. No blood samples need to be taken except for initial calibration. The advantages of a continuous on-line display of $SjvO_2$ are easily apparent. This technique, however, does have its disadvantages. Calibration drift may occur and frequent in vivo recalibration may be required. Inaccurate readings can be obtained if the sensor is impacted against the vessel wall or if there is a decrease in intensity of the near infrared light in the fibreoptic sensor which occurs with thrombus formation on the catheter tip, changes in head position or blood flow characteristics in the vein.

FACTORS AFFECTING $SjvO_2$

Although $SjvO_2$ does not give quantitative information about either CBF or $CMRO_2$, it reflects the balance between the two variables. Reductions in $SjvO_2$ or increases in $AJDO_2$ below 9 ml/dl provide useful markers for inadequate CBF. Causes of altered $SjvO_2$ are given in Figure 53.2.

The threshold of $SjvO_2$ below which cerebral ischaemia occurs may vary with the individual and the pathology. The two most common causes of jugular bulb desaturation ($SjvO_2$ < 55%) are:

1. *Decreased CPP* due to raised ICP or systemic hypotension.
2. *Hypocapnia*: In head-injured patients, $SjvO_2$ values less than 50% have been shown to increase mortality.[1] In patients undergoing cardiopulmonary bypass for cardiac surgery, cerebral venous desaturation below 50% correlated with worse postoperative cognitive function.[2]

CLINICAL APPLICATIONS

A rise in ICP associated with a normal or low $SjvO_2$ would suggest that oedema is the predominant cause. If ICP and $SjvO_2$ were both high, hyperaemia would be implicated and hyperventilation the appropriate therapy $SjvO_2$ may therefore help target appropriate therapy.

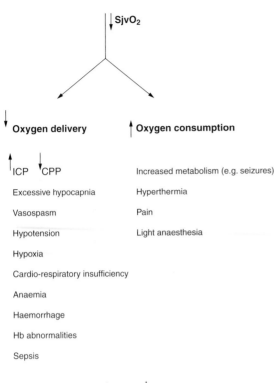

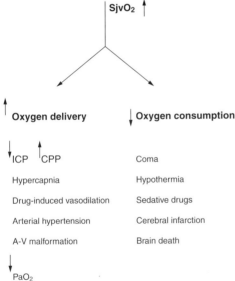

Figure 53.2   Factors affecting SjvO$_2$

There are also benefits in measuring SjvO$_2$ to assess cerebral hypoperfusion during the perioperative management of patients with SAH.

CMRO$_2$ can be calculated using the equation:
CMRO$_2$ = CBF × (SaO$_2$ − SjO$_2$).

Assuming haemoglobin concentration is the same in arterial and venous blood and the amount of dissolved oxygen is minimal, arteriojugular oxygen content difference can be substituted for arteriojugular oxygen saturation difference. Hence:

CMRO$_2$ = CBF × (SaO$_2$ − SjvO$_2$).

LIMITATIONS

The main limitation of this form of monitoring is that it is a *global* measure and a regional change in cerebral oxygenation will not be detected unless it is of sufficient magnitude to affect overall brain saturation. It is, however, the most widely used monitor for cerebral oxygenation in neuroanaesthesia and intensive care.

KEY POINTS

- SjvO$_2$ is a global measure of the balance of CBF and CMRO$_2$.
- Insertion technique and complications are similar to an internal jugular central venous line.
- Measurement can be intermittent or continuous.
- Measurement of SjvO$_2$ is useful in monitoring interventions such as hyperventilation therapy.
- Lack of sensitivity to regional changes is a major limitation.

FURTHER READING

Feldman Z, Robertson CS. Monitoring of cerebral hemodynamics with jugular bulb catheters. Crit Care Clin 1997; 13: 51–77

Dearden NM, Midgley S. Technical considerations in continuous jugular venous oxygen saturation measurement. Acta Neurochir 1993; 59 (Suppl): 91–97

Gupta AK, Bullock MR. Monitoring the injured brain in the intensive care unit: present and future. Hospital Med 1998; 59 (9): 704–713

Robertson CS, Gopinath SP, Goodman JC, Contant CF, Valadka AB, Narayan RK. SjvO$_2$ monitoring in head injured patients. J Neurotrauma 1995; 12: 891–896

REFERENCES

1. Sheinberg M, Kanter MJ, Robertson CS, Constant CF, Narayan RK, Grossman RG. Continuous monitoring

SjvO$_2$ is a useful technique to guide hyperventilation therapy. Excessive hyperventilation causes profound cerebral vasoconstriction, which results in a reduction of SjvO$_2$, assuming brain metabolism remains constant. SjvO$_2$ should be kept above 55% if hyperventilation is instituted.

of jugular venous oxygen saturation in head-injured patients. J Neurosurg 1992; 76: 212–271

2. Croughwell ND, White WD, Smith LR, Davis RD, Glower DD, Reeves JG, Newman MF. Jugular bulb saturation and mixed venous saturation during cardiopulmonary bypass. J Card Surg 1995; 10: 503–508

54

NEAR INFRARED
SPECTROSCOPY

A.K. Gupta

INTRODUCTION

Near infrared spectroscopy (NIRS) is a non-invasive method of estimating *regional* cerebral oxygenation.

The physical principles behind NIRS are based upon the fact that light in the near infrared red range (700–1000 nm) can pass through skin, bone and other tissues relatively easily. When a beam of light is passed through brain tissue, it is both *scattered* and *absorbed*. The absorption of near infrared light is proportional to the concentration of certain chromophores, notably iron in haemoglobin and copper in cytochrome aa_3. Oxygenated (HbO_2), deoxygenated haemoglobin (Hb) and cytochrome aa_3 have different absorption spectra, and the concentration of each depends on the substances' oxygenation status. The isobestic point of HbO_2 and Hb is at about 810 nm. Oxyhaemoglobin has a greater light absorption above this wavelength and deoxyhaemoglobin has greater light absorption below 810nm. The maximum light absorption of cytochrome aa_3, which is the terminal member of the mitochondrial respiratory chain, is at 830 mm. Measurement of absorption at a number of wavelengths provides an estimate of oxidation status (see below).

Changes of concentration of near infrared light as it passes through these compounds can be quantified using a modified Beer-Lambert law which describes optical attenuation. It is expressed as:

$$\text{Attenuation (OD)} = \text{Log} \frac{Ia}{I} \alpha\, LB + G$$

where OD = Optical density, Ia = Incident light intensity, I = Detected light intensity, α = Absorption coefficient of chromophore (mM^{-1} cm^{-1}), C = Concentration of chromophore (mM), L = Distance between the points where light enters and leaves the tissue (cm), B = Pathlength factor, G = Factor related to the measurement geometry and type of tissue.

NIRS is ideally suited to infants because of the thinness of the skull. Changes in absorption can be measured for light transmitted from one side of the skull and detected on the opposite side (*Transmission spectroscopy*). In adults, NIRS measurement cannot be made by transillumination because of the diameter of the head and thickness of the skull which causes significant attenuation. Reflected light is therefore measured (*reflectance spectroscopy*) (Fig. 54.1).

EQUIPMENT

Near infrared instruments are made for clinical use by a number of manufacturers. Light is generated at up to four different wavelengths by laser photodiodes and detected by a silicon photodiode. The light sources are recessed so as to prevent direct skin contact.

The probes illuminate up to a volume of 10 ml of hemispherical tissue. The radial depth depends on the interoptode distance. The optodes are placed on one side of the forehead away from the midline, cerebral venous sinuses, temporalis muscle and at an acute angle to each other with an interrupted spacing of 4–7 cm (Fig. 54.1).

Using a derived algorithm the measured changes in attenuation at each wavelength (for each chromophore) can be converted into equivalent changes in the concentration of HbO_2, Hb and cytochrome aa_3. All measurements are expressed as absolute concentration *changes* from an arbitrary zero at the start of the measurement period. Normal values of HbO_2 are reported to be 60–80%.

CLINICAL APPLICATION

In neonates, NIRS can give an absolute measure of changing brain haemoglobin saturation and blood volume and provides a means of monitoring the cerebrovascular response to certain therapeutic manipulations. In adults, NIRS has been used to monitor patients with head injury, SAH, and patients undergoing carotid endarterectomy (CEA).

- *CEA*: Cerebral desaturation on ICA cross-clamping has been observed in more than 50% of patients which was reversed either by release of cross-clamping or placement of an intraoperative shunt. As part of the multimodal monitoring system, NIRS helps identify patients who require intraoperative shunting.

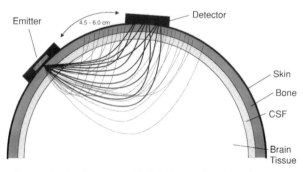

Figure 54.1   Principle of NIRS. (Reproduced with permission from Al-Rawi.)

- *Head injury:* Various studies have demonstrated that desaturations in patients with HI on the ICU seem to correlate well with SjvO₂, laser Doppler flowmetry and TCD. However, the NIRS changes do not always match SjvO₂. Practical difficulties in maintaining the sensor position long-term are a major problem for this application.
- *Cardiopulmonary bypass (CPB):* Changes in oxygenation have been investigated but the effects of CPB on the assumptions made in the algorithm have not been fully evaluated.
- *Cerebral blood flow* has been estimated using NIRS by using HbO₂ as a tracer and calculating CBF using a modification of the Fick principle.
- *Cerebral blood volume* has been estimated by various investigators with NIRS to measure changes in *total* Hb or changes in HbO₂ vs SpO₂.

ADVANTAGES OVER OTHER TECHNIQUES

- NIRS is a *regional* indicator of cerebral oxygenation, whereas SjvO₂ is more *global*. It has the advantage of being non-invasive. SjvO₂ is invasive, has no spatial resolution and is prone to error for a number of reasons (see Chapter 53).
- NIRS has the advantage over laser-Doppler flowmetry in that it is non-invasive, is less prone to movement artefact and probe placement over large surface vessels.
- Although TCD ultrasound is portable and non-invasive it can only measure blood flow velocity in large cerebral arteries and extracranial vessels and does not give information about oxygenation of tissues.
- Near infrared technology does not use ionising radiation, is portable and provides continuous readings with a high temporal resolution. This is in contrast to imaging techniques such as PET, SPECT or Xenon-133.

DISADVANTAGES

- Although a non-invasive method of measuring CBF and CBV would be advantageous, significant variability still exists between NIRS measurements and 'gold standard' measurements such as Xenon washout or PET.
- One of the major problems that still exists with this technology is the inability to reliably distinguish between intra- and extracranial changes in blood flow and oxygenation. Extracranial contamination of the measured signal adversely affects the reliability of the readings.

- Optode separation will affect the degree of extracranial contamination, which decreases with increased optode spacing. Excessive distance will lead to a very weak signal. It is accepted that the optimal distance between optodes is 4–7 cm.
- Different equipment may use different algorithms.
- Pathlength factor may change in various situations and is wavelength-dependent.
- NIRS machines have reduced in size over the last few years but still remain quite bulky. The signal is sensitive to outside light and head movement will also affect the recording.
- The readings are regional and the amount of intracranial tissue monitored is variable depending on interoptode spacing. To allow a truly multiregional monitoring system, multiple probes would be required.

Regardless of these problems, however, NIRS is able to monitor trends in oxygenation in the individual patient and may be useful as an adjunct to a multimodal monitoring system.

KEY POINTS

- NIRS is a non-invasive method of measuring regional cerebral oxygenation.
- It measures changes in the differential absorption of certain chromophores (HbO₂, Hb, cyt aa₃).
- Its use has been demonstrated intraoperatively and in ICU.
- The main problem with the reliability of the readings is the relative contribution of extracerebral blood flow.
- The distance between the optodes is ideally between 4 and 7 cm.

FURTHER READING

Harris DNF, Bailey SM. Near infrared spectroscopy in adults. Anaesthesia 1993; 48: 694–696

Kirkpatrick PJ, Smielewski P, Whitfield P, Czosnyka M, Menon D, Pickard J. An observational study of near infrared spectroscopy during carotid endarterectomy. J Neurosurg 1995; 82: 756–763

Owen-Reece H, Smith M, Elwell CE, Goldstone JC. Near infrared spectroscopy. Br J Anaes 1999; 82: 418–426

Kirkpatrick PJ, Smielewski P, Czosnyka M, Menon DK, Pickard JD. Near infrared spectroscopy use in patients with head injury. J Neurosurg 1995; 83: 963–970

Gupta AK, Menon DK, Czosnyka M, Smielewski P, Kirkpatrick PJ, Jones JG. Non-invasive measurement of cerebral blood volume in volunteers. Br J Anaes 1997; 78: 39–43

Germon TJ, Young AER, Alexander R, Manara AR, Nelson RJ. Extracerebral absorption of near infrared light influences the detection of increased cerebral oxygenation monitored by near infrared spectroscopy. J Neurol Neurosurg Psychiatry 1995; 58: 477–479

55

MEASUREMENT OF TISSUE OXYGENATION

A.K. Gupta

INTRODUCTION

Measurement of cerebral oxygenation is an integral part of the management of patients with brain injury. Although the ability to measure oxygen tension in tissue was first reported by Clark in 1956, the most established method of monitoring cerebral oxygenation clinically is using jugular bulb oximetry (see Chapter 53). More recently, sensors have been implanted into brain tissue as a measure of cerebral oxygenation and metabolism. This may be of use in:

1. The early detection of secondary insults so that interventions can be made to prevent further ischaemia.
2. Optimisation of oxygen delivery to areas of marginal perfusion.
3. Monitoring the well-being of uninjured areas of brain.
4. Guiding therapy.
5. Understanding the mechanisms causing secondary injury.

PRINCIPLES AND EQUIPMENT

At present two commercially available sensors are used:

- *Licox sensor* (GMS, Germany) which measures brain tissue oxygen tension,
- *Neurotrend sensor* (Codman, USA) which measures brain tissue oxygen, CO_2 and pH (PbO_2, $PbCO_2$ and pHb).

Both of these methods have the ability to measure brain temperature, are approximately 0.5 mm in diameter and are calibrated prior to insertion.

The *Licox* system consists of a sensor which includes a polarographic electrochemical microsensor that measures oxygen and a thermocouple for temperature measurement. The probes come with an application system which includes a bolt that can be fixed into the skull. A raw signal is generated by the reduction of oxygen after diffusing from tissue through the polyethylene wall of the catheter tube into its inner electrolyte chamber. The sensor is connected to a monitor which displays values of PO_2 and temperature.

The *Neurotrend* is made up of four different sensors staggered over approximately 2 cm (Fig. 55.1). The oxygen sensor consists of a fibre in which the holes are filled with silicone rubber that contains entrapped ruthenium-based dye. Blue light at 450–470 nm is passed down the fibre which is absorbed by the dye. The dye emits a proportion of the energy it has absorbed as light of another wavelength, in this case 620 nm. In the presence of oxygen, however, the amount of this fluorescent light is reduced, so-called 'oxygen quenching'. The amount of quenching is proportional to the concentration of oxygen and thus, if the amount of fluorescent light is measured an estimation of the oxygen concentration can be made.

The pH and CO_2 sensors both contain phenol red dye which changes colour in response to the concentration of hydrogen ions and changes the absorption of green light. The CO_2 sensor is similar to the pH fibre with the addition of a gas-permeable membrane enclosing the holes in the fibre. Only CO_2 can pass through the membrane which changes the pH of a surrounding bicarbonate solution which is detected by the change in dye colour. The change is reversible so that both increases and decreases in pH can be detected by irradiating the dye cell with green light. A thermocouple and the three sensors are placed inside a polyethylene sheath.

CLINICAL APPLICATIONS

These sensors have been primarily used in patients with severe HI and poor grade SAH both in intensive

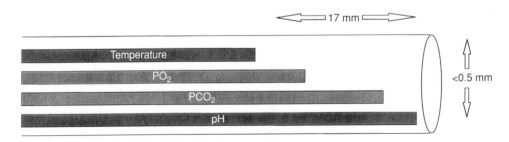

Figure 55.1   Diagrammatic representation of a cross section of the Neurotrend™ sensor. (Reproduced with permission from Codman UK.)

care and in the operating room. Tissue PO_2 (PbO_2) is normally lower than arterial PaO_2 due to the extravascular sensor placement and high metabolic activity of the brain (range 15–50 mmHg); $PbCO_2$ is normally higher than $PaCO_2$ and is directly related, reflecting the high diffusibility of CO_2 (range 40–70 mmHg); pH is normally lower in brain tissue (pHb), also reflecting high brain metabolism (range 7.05–7.25).

Head injury

PbO_2 tension is generally lower in HI, with reported values < 10 mmHg. Demonstrable rises in $PbCO_2$ and concomitant falls PbO_2 and pHb occur during brain death. Changes in these parameters have been shown to be different in normal and abnormal areas of brain. These sensors are useful in monitoring changes in *trends* of cerebral oxygenation, detecting secondary insults and guiding specific therapy such as hyperventilation and induced hypothermia.

Subarachnoid haemorrhage

Profound changes in all parameters have been shown in various studies with prolonged temporary clipping of feeder vessels during surgery. This has correlated well with changes in brain chemistry using microdialysis (see Chapter 56, Fig. 56.2). An example of the

effects of temporary clipping on brain tissue parameters of O_2, CO_2 tension and pH is shown in Figure 55.2.

RESPONSE TO PHYSIOLOGICAL VARIABLES

Reduction in PbO_2 as a result of arterial desaturation has been demonstrated by numerous authors. In head-injured patients a rise in PbO_2 occurs in response to increased inspired O_2. A correlation between PbO_2 and regional CBF has been reported. Tissue CO_2 and pH seem to change in parallel with arterial CO_2 and pH except in ischaemia when $PbCO_2$ increases and pHb decreases.

SAFETY AND VALIDATION

There have been many reports of the use of these sensors in both animal and human studies with no reports of any major complications to date. Stable and reproducible results have been published which correlate with *in vitro* methods. Changes in PbO_2 have been shown to correlate well with changes in $SjvO_2$ and end capillary PO_2 measured by positron emission tomography.

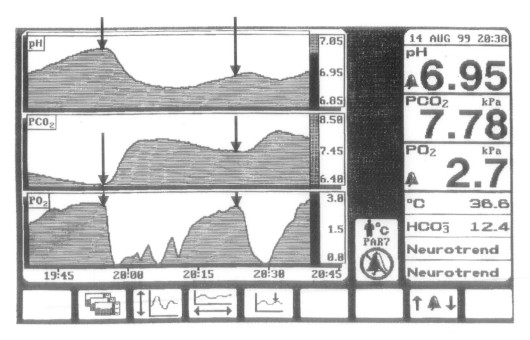

Figure 55.2   Tracing from a Neurotrend ™ monitor showing changes in brain tissue PO_2, PCO_2 and pH as a result of temporary clip application of an artery feeding an MCA aneurysm shown by the arrows. (Reproduced with permission from R. Kett-White.) PbO_2 decreases to 0 after both episodes of temporary clipping. Tissue CO_2 rises and pH falls after the first episode of clipping. Tissue O_2 recovers when the clip is removed

ADVANTAGES OF TISSUE MONITORING

- Enables a continuous method of monitoring.
- Regional changes can be detected.
- Readings are more reliable and technically easier to maintain than continuous jugular venous oximetry.
- Allows selective monitoring of tissue with marginal perfusion.
- Allows direct monitoring of brain temperature.

DISADVANTAGES OF TISSUE MONITORING

- It is an invasive technique with associated risks.
- The sensors are very fragile.
- It does not reflect global changes.
- More data is required to confirm clinical usefulness.

KEY POINTS

- New technology enables measurement of brain tissue PO_2, PCO_2 pH and temperature.
- Changes in brain oxygenation have been demonstrated in patients with HI and SAH.

- Although invasive, no major complications have been reported with this technique to date.
- Further data are being accumulated regarding the clinical utility of these sensors.
- They may become an integral part of the multi-modal monitoring system of the injured brain in the future.

FURTHER READING

Dings J, Meixensberger J, Roosen K. Brain tissue PO_2 monitoring: catheter stability and complications. Neurol Res 1997; 19: 241–245

Gupta AK, Hutchinson PJ, Al-Rawi P, et al. Measurement of brain tissue oxygenation compared with jugular venous oxygen saturation for monitoring cerebral oxygenation after traumatic brain injury. Anes Anal 1999; 88(3): 549–553

Hutchinson PJ, Al-Rawi P, O'Connel MT, et al. Monitoring of brain metabolism during aneurysm surgery using microdialysis and brain multiparameter sensors. Neurol Res 1999; 21: 352–358

Santbrink H, Maas AIR, Avezaat CJJ. Continuous monitoring of partial pressure of brain tissue oxygen in patients with severe head injury. Neurosurgery 1996; 38: 21–31

Zauner A, Bullock R, Di X, Young HF. Brain oxygen CO_2 pH and temperature monitoring: Evaluation in the feline brain. J Neurosurg 1995; 37: 1168–1177

56

MICRODIALYSIS

P. J. A. Hutchinson

INTRODUCTION

Microdialysis is a technique which monitors the chemistry of body tissues and organs directly. Human cerebral microdialysis was introduced in the early 1990s and has been applied to the investigation of head injury, subarachnoid haemorrhage, epilepsy and tumours.

A fine catheter, approximately 0.5 mm in diameter, lined with dialysis membrane is placed within the cerebral cortex and perfused with a physiological solution at ultra-low flow rates (0.1–2.0 μl/min). Substrate and metabolite molecules, (e.g. glucose, pyruvate, lactate, glutamate and glycerol), diffuse from the extracellular space across the membrane into the solution which is then collected for biochemical analysis (Fig. 56.1).

The ability to measure the concentration of molecules in the extracellular space of the brain has the potential to provide a monitor of patient progress during injury or illness and to increase understanding of the pathophysiology of disease.

EQUIPMENT

The microdialysis equipment comprises a fine concentric catheter, lined with dialysis membrane attached to a syringe of perfusion fluid such as normal saline or Ringer's solution in an ultra-low flow rate pump. Fluid passes from the syringe via an inlet tube to the catheter where dialysis occurs and exits from the catheter via an outlet tube connected to collecting vials. These vials are changed at set intervals of between 10 and 60 minutes. Chemical analysis is ideally performed using automated on line bedside enzymatic analysers. Samples can then be frozen for

later analysis of more complex molecules using high performance liquid chromatography.

The microdialysis catheter can be placed into the brain directly through a burrhole and tunnelled under the scalp or inserted via a bolt in conjunction with other probes (e.g. intracranial pressure and multi-parameter tissue gas sensors, see Chapter 55). The catheter can be located in areas of uninjured brain or in the region of ischaemia as defined by imaging. Simultaneous peripheral microdialysis can be performed in subcutaneous adipose tissue of the anterior abdominal wall to correlate cerebral changes with systemic chemistry.

CRITICAL APPRAISAL

The main concern using invasive probes is local implantation trauma. This is minimised by using very fine catheters (0.5 mm). Studies in animals and man have demonstrated that the blood–brain barrier remains intact with very little evidence of neuro-pathological change.

When applying microdialysis clinically, there is always a compromise between low flow rates (to increase the relative recovery rates) and high flow rates (to increase the volume of dialysate available for analysis).

True extracellular concentrations of substances may not be measured if full equilibration does not occur at the site of the membrane. It can, however, be determined by *in vivo* recovery studies including:

1. The no net flux technique (applying varying concentrations of the substance of interest to the dialysis fluid and determining the concentration that does not change following equilibration).
2. The extrapolation to zero flow method (varying the flow rate and extrapolating to zero flow to determine the concentration that would exist in the presence of zero flow after complete equilibration).

CLINICAL APPLICATIONS

Cerebral microdialysis has been applied to patients in intensive care and the operating room.

Head injury

Derangements in metabolism associated with reductions in brain glucose and elevation of the lactate:pyruvate ratio have been demonstrated during periods of intracranial hypertension and cerebral ischaemia. Wide variations in the concentration of

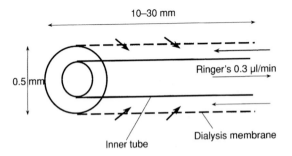

Figure 56.1   Diagram of a concentric microdialysis catheter consisting of two tubes. Physiological solution is pumped between the space of the outer tube of dialysis membrane and the inner tube. Molecules diffuse across the membrane from extracellular fluid into the physiological solution and on reaching the tip of the catheter, pass up the inner tube into collecting vials for analysis

the excitatory amino acids glutamate and aspartate have also been detected, with extremely high levels in secondary ischaemia and contusions.

Subarachnoid Haemorrhage

During aneurysm surgery, changes in concentration of glucose, lactate, pyruvate and glutamate have been demonstrated during CSF drainage, brain retraction and temporary clipping. The combination of micro-dialysis and multiparameter sensors can monitor the effect of clinical events on brain metabolism (Fig. 56.2). The chemistry of ventilated patients with poor grade SAH on the intensive care unit can also be assessed.

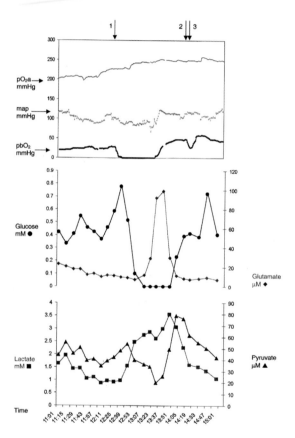

Figure 56.2 Perioperative mean arterial blood pressure (MAP), arterial oxygen (pO₂a), brain oxygen (pO₂b), and microdialysis parameters in a patient undergoing aneurysm clipping. Arrow 1 indicates a decrease in (pO₂b) associated with mild hypotension (measured using an intraparenchymal multiparameter sensor – Paratrend). This was accompanied by decreases in glucose and pyruvate and increases in lactate and glutamate. Arrow 2 indicates a second decrease in (pO₂b) due to hydrocephalus which recovered on re-opening the dura (arrow 3). (Reproduced with permission from Hutchinson et al. Neurosurgery 2000; 46: 201–206.)

Epilepsy

Epileptic foci in the temporal lobe are associated with elevated glutamate and reduced γ-amino-butyric acid levels prior to seizures and increases in both amino acids during seizures.

Tumours

By implanting the microdialysis catheter directly into gliomas, chemotherapeutic agents can be added to the perfusion fluid and delivered to the centre of the tumour.

KEY POINTS

- Microdialysis directly measures the concentration of substrates and metabolites in the extracellular space including substances such as glucose, pyruvate, lactate and neurotransmitters.
- It is presently used as a research technique to monitor the progress of the injured brain and to increase understanding of disease processes.

FURTHER READING

Editorial: Microdialysis. Lancet 1992; 339: 1326–1327

Hutchinson PJA, Al-Rawi PG, O'Connell MT, et al. Monitoring of brain metabolism during aneurysm surgery using microdialysis and brain multiparameter sensors. Neurol Res 1999; 21: 352–358

Mendelowitsch A, Sekhar LN, Wright DC, et al. An increase in extracellular glutamate is a sensitive method of detecting ischaemic neuronal damage during cranial base and cerebrovascular surgery. An in vivo microdialysis study. Acta Neurochir Wien 1998; 140: 349–355

Persson L, Valtysson J, Enblad P, et al. Neurochemical monitoring using intracerebral microdialysis in patients with subarachnoid haemorrhage. J Neurosurg 1996; 84: 606–616

Robertson CS, Gopinath SP, Uzura M, Valadka AB, Goodman JC. Metabolic changes in the brain during transient ischemia measured with microdialysis. Neurol Res 1998; 20 (Suppl 1): S91–S94

Ungerstedt U. Microdialysis-principles and applications for studies in animals and man. J Intern Med 1991; 230: 365–373

Vespa P, Prins M, Ronne-Engstrom E, et al. Increase in extracellular glutamate caused by reduced cerebral perfusion pressure and seizures after traumatic brain injury: a microdialysis study. J Neurosurg 1998; 89: 971–982

Whittle IR. Intracerebral microdialysis: a new method in applied clinical neuroscience research. Br J Neurosurg 1990; 4: 459–462

57

EVOKED POTENTIAL AND PERIPHERAL NEUROPHYSIOLOGY

B. McNamara

INTRODUCTION

Evoked potentials are the electrical response of the cerebral cortex, subcortical nuclei, brainstem and spinal cord to a peripheral sensory stimulus. Nerve conduction studies (NCS) and EMG are used to examine the peripheral nervous system.

EVOKED POTENTIALS

The most commonly used are the visual evoked potential (VEP) which is the response of the occipital cortex to a visual stimulus (normally a flash or a reversing checkerboard), the brainstem auditory evoked potential (BAEP) which is the response of brainstem nuclei to a simple auditory stimulus and the somatosensory evoked potential (SEP) which is the response of the cerebral cortex and spinal cord to peripheral sensory stimulation (normally electrical stimulation of a sensory or mixed peripheral nerve). These responses are quite small when compared with background electrical activity and to improve resolution of the response the average response to a large number of stimuli is produced.

SOMATOSENSORY EVOKED POTENTIALS (SEP)

The upper limb SEP is produced by electrical stimulation of the median or ulnar nerve. The lower limb SEP is produced by electrical stimulation of the posterior tibial nerve. The cortical and spinal cord responses are summarised in Figure 57.1. The spinal recorded response is generated by dorsal horn interneurones (P15), the first cortical recorded response (N20) is generated by the posterior bank of the rolandic fissure.

Clinical Applications

Measurement of peak latency and peak-to-peak amplitude of the SEP is a particularly useful means of monitoring spinal cord and brain function during surgery.

Spinal surgery

Cortical SEP or spinal SEP recorded using epidural electrodes are particularly useful for protecting the spinal cord during surgery. Indirect evidence shows that SEP monitoring during scoliosis surgery reduces the incidence of operative morbidity.

Carotid surgery

A fall in CBF of >30% will result in a decline in SEP amplitude. Monitoring the cortical components of

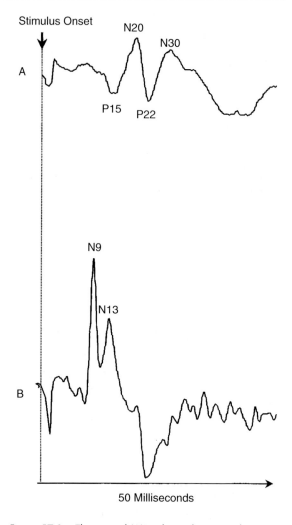

Figure 57.1   The cortical (A) and spinal SEP (B). The principal cortical components (N20/P22) are generated by the primary somatosensory cortex. The N9 component of the spinal SEP is generated in the brachial plexus while the N13 is generated in the dorsal column and dorsal horn

the SEP is a useful alternative to EEG monitoring in carotid surgery.

Aneurysm surgery

Limitations to blood flow during aneurysm surgery can be detected using SEPs, particularly involving the anterior cerebral circulation.

Postoperative care and ICU

The SEP is a useful means of predicting outcome in post-traumatic and anoxic patients. There is good evidence demonstrating that a bilaterally absent SEP is strongly associated with a very poor outcome.

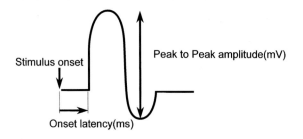

Figure 57.2 Measured characteristics of the compound motor action potential (CMAP). To calculate the motor conduction velocity (MCV) the nerve is stimulated distally and proximally, the velocity can then be calculated using the following: MCV = Distance between stimulation points (mm)/(Proximal latency-Distal latency(ms))

Continuous bilateral SEP monitoring is a useful means of detecting the development of cerebral ischaemia in at-risk patients.

OTHER EVOKED POTENTIALS

VEPs may be used to monitor optic nerve function during pituitary gland surgery or surgery in the anterior cranial fossa. Brainstem evoked responses are sometimes used for monitoring during posterior craniotomy such as resection of acoustic neuroma, other cerebellopontine angle tumours or in microvascular decompression for trigeminal neuralgia.

Anaesthetic Effects

Anaesthetics minimally affect BAEPs and spinal recorded SEPs. Cortical SEPs and VEPs are very sensitive to inhalational anaesthetics including N_2O, giving a dose-dependent increase in latency and decrease in amplitude. The evoked potential is usually abolished above 1 MAC.

Large bolus doses of intravenous agents have similar effects without actually abolishing the potential.

Motor evoked potentials are more sensitive to anaesthetic agents with a very variable response. They also require the absence of significant amounts of muscle relaxants.

Temperature changes, either systemic or locally along any point in the conduction pathway will also affect latency and amplitude.

NERVE CONDUCTION STUDIES

Motor nerve conduction studies involve stimulating a motor nerve or mixed nerve with a supra-maximal electrical stimulus at two or more points along its course. The response is then recorded from a distal muscle innervated by the tested nerve. The response recorded is known as the compound motor action potential (CMAP) (Fig. 57.2), the CMAP is generated by the action potentials of a large number of muscle fibres. Measurements of latency and amplitude of this response can give useful information about the motor conduction velocity and the number of intact motor fibres.

Sensory nerve conduction studies are performed by stimulating the nerve using a supramaximal electrical stimulus and then recording the compound sensory action potential (SAP). The recorded response is generated by the action potentials of many individual nerve fibres. Measurements of the latency and amplitude of this response can allow the sensory conduction velocity to be calculated and can give an indication of the number of intact sensory fibres (Fig. 57.3).

Mixed nerve conduction studies are performed by stimulating the nerve trunk of a mixed nerve proximally and recording the compound nerve action potential proximally.

The F wave is a late CMAP produced by the backfiring of antidromically activated motor neurones (Fig. 57.4). The H reflex is an electrically evoked monosynaptic reflex.

EMG

EMG is an examination of the electrical activity produced by a muscle. It is usually performed by inserting a concentric needle electrode into the muscle to be examined, this consists of an outer stainless steel cannula which acts as the reference electrode and an inner wire which acts as the recording electrode. During a typical EMG examination the spontaneous activity, the activity of the muscle fibres innervated by a single motor unit (motor unit action potentials), and activation at maximal recruitment are all examined.

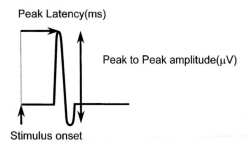

Figure 57.3 Measured characteristics of the sensory action potential. Sensory conduction velocity (SCV) can be calculated using the following: SCV = Distance between stimulation and recording electrodes (mm)/Latency(ms)

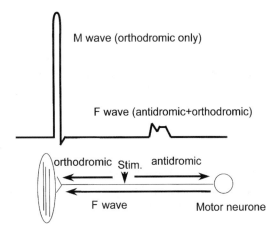

Figure 57.4   The F wave. The M wave is produced by normal orthodromic stimulation of the motor nerve. In addition an antidromic impulse travels to the anterior horn cell which is then stimulated to produce a later, smaller response – the F wave. The F wave is a useful means of assessing the proximal portions of the nerve

Clinical Applications

Nerve conduction studies can be used to diagnose and classify generalised neuropathies (e.g. to differentiate between axonal neuropathies such as the diabetic neuropathies and demyelinating neuropathies).

In axonal neuropathies the amplitude of sensory and motor responses falls but conduction velocities are well preserved. In demyelinating neuropathies the amplitude of the responses may fall but in addition the conduction velocity is reduced and there may also be a significant fall in CMAP amplitude on proximal stimulation (motor conduction block) and dispersion of the response.

Nerve conduction studies are also an essential part of the preoperative assessment of entrapment neuropathies (e.g. carpal tunnel syndrome and ulnar nerve entrapment at the elbow). They can confirm the diagnosis, give an indication of the severity and allow the site of entrapment to be precisely localised.

Facial nerve monitoring is a useful means of protecting the facial nerve during surgery which is particularly useful in cerebello-pontine angle surgery and parotid surgery.

EMG can be useful in the diagnosis of anterior horn cell disease, nerve root and plexus lesions, neuropathies and primary muscle diseases. EMG and nerve conduction studies may also be a useful adjunct to imaging in the diagnosis of nerve root entrapment and plexus lesions. Nerve conduction studies and EMG are important means of diagnosing neuromuscular disease in the ICU (Table 57.1).

TRANSCRANIAL/CERVICAL MAGNETIC STIMULATION

The sensory evoked potentials (SEP, BAEP and VEP) examine afferent pathways only. The brain, spinal cord and peripheral nerves can be stimulated by a magnetic pulse delivered using a coil placed on the skin surface and the muscular response may be

Condition	Motor NCS	Sensory NCS	F waves	EMG
Table 57.1 Some neuromuscular conditions causing respiratory failure and the findings found on nerve conduction studies and EMG				
Guillain–Barré syndrome	Slowing of conduction, Conduction block	SAP may be reduced or absent	Delayed or absent	May show late dennervation
Motor neurone disease	Reduced CMAP amplitude but velocity at least 70% of normal	Normal	Normal when CMAP amplitudes normal	Widespread dennervation
Myositis	Reduced with acceptable velocity	Normal	Normal	Myopathic features
Myasthenia gravis	Reduced CMAP with decrement on repetitive stimulation	Normal	Normal	Increased jitter on single fibre EMG

measured electrically. This can be used as an alternative to SEP to ensure the integrity of the spinal cord during spinal cord surgery.

KEY POINTS

- Evoked potentials are the electrical response of the brain to a peripheral sensory stimulus.
- SEP measurements may be used to monitor spinal cord function during spinal surgery and brain function during carotid and aneurysm surgery.
- Nerve conduction studies and EMG are useful means of diagnosing neuromuscular disease in the ICU. They are also useful for the preoperative assessment of entrapment neuropathies and radiculopathies.
- Transcranial and trans-cervical magnetic stimulation can be used to assess diaphragmatic function and cortico-diaphragmatic pathways.

FURTHER READING

Jones SJ. Evoked potentials in intraoperative monitoring. In: Halliday AM (ed.) Evoked potentials in clinical testing. London: Churchill Livingstone, 1993

Sethi RK, Thompson LL. The electromyographer's handbook. Boston: Little Brown, 1989

58

ELECTROENCEPHALOGRAPHY AND CEREBRAL FUNCTION MONITORING

B. McNamara

INTRODUCTION

An EEG represents spontaneous electrical activity of the cerebral cortex. It is generated mainly by summation of excitatory and inhibitory post-synaptic potentials of cortical neurones and recorded from scalp electrodes attached via viscous conducting gel rich in AgCl ions. These electrodes are arranged on the surface of the scalp according to a standard electrode placement system – the 10–20 Electrode System based on a series of lines from key landmarks drawn over the scalp (nasion to inion, left to right aural tragus, midfrontal and midparietal lobes; Fig. 58.1). A letter prefix designates brain site (i.e. C = central, F = frontal, P = parietal, T = temporal). Numbers indicate relative distance from the midline (nasion to inion). Right-sided electrodes are given even numbers, odd numbers to the left and midline electrodes are designated 'Z', e.g. T3 is the left temporal side; CZ is the central midline.

Electrical activity is either recorded between pairs of electrodes or between each electrode and a common reference point. The electrical signal is amplified, filtered (removing unwanted electrical signals from sources such as EMG, movement and radiofrequency) and then displayed as either 8 or 16 channels (8 channels per hemisphere) to give an accurate representation of electrical activity throughout the cortex. The EEG represents electrical activity over the cerebral cortex only and does not reflect activity in subcortical levels, cranial nerves or the spinal cord.

EEG activity is usually interpreted in terms of:

1. *Frequency*: Activity is usually grouped into one of four frequency bands: δ (< 4 Hz), θ (4–8 Hz), α (8–13 Hz) and β (> 13 Hz) (Fig. 58.2).
2. *Amplitude*: Most EEG activity is between 20 and 200 μV.
3. *Location*: Multi-channel EEG determines whether the electrical activity is localised or generated throughout the cortex.

Normal awake adults show symmetrical rhythm of approximately 9 Hz (α rhythm) located posteriorly toward the occipital lobes and attenuated when the eyes are open, i.e. a desynchronised EEG with irregular low voltage activity without a dominant frequency. Certain neurological conditions are characterised by paroxysmal abnormal activity, e.g. the spikes or sharp waves of epilepsy.

AUTOMATED EEG PROCESSING

To facilitate continuous EEG monitoring several automated EEG processing systems have been developed.

1. *Power spectral analysis*: This is a frequency-based method. The signal is mathematically manipulated by fast Fourier transformation of small intervals of EEG to provide a graphical representation of the relative power content of the various frequency bands in each segment of EEG (Fig. 58.3; power = voltage^2/resistance). These spectral diagrams are then stacked to show how the frequency of the EEG alters with time to produce a compressed

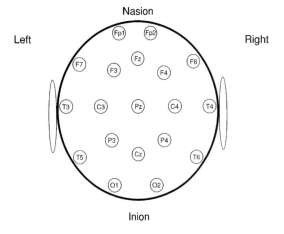

Figure 58.1   The international 10–20 system of EEG electrode placement. F = frontal, C = central, P = parietal, T = temporal, O = occipital. Right-sided placements are indicated by even numbers, left-sided placements by odd numbers and midline placements by Z

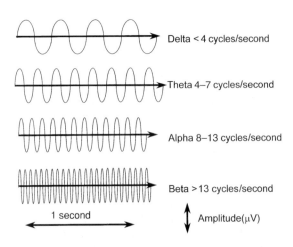

Figure 58.2   Most EEG activity is defined in terms of frequency and amplitude. A schematic diagram of the four frequency bands is shown above

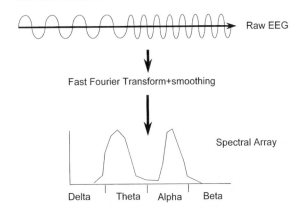

Figure 58.3 Spectral array, the digitised EEG signal is mathematically transformed to produce a spectral array showing the distribution of frequencies in that segment of EEG

Table 58.1 BIS range guidelines	
BIS	**Hypnotic state**
100	Awake Light to moderate sedation
70	Light hypnotic state Low probability of explicit recall < 70
60	Moderate hypnotic state Low probability of consciousness < 60
40	Deep hypnotic state
0	EEG suppression

spectral array. This spectral analysis can also give a single number (either the mean frequency or the frequency below which 95% of the signal lies) that can be tracked over time.

3. *Cerebral function monitor (CFM):* This provides a single trace of total power varying with both amplitude and frequency of raw EEG data. Because only a single trace is produced this may be more easily interpreted.

3. *Cerebral function analysing monitor (CFAM):* A similar method, which produces displays of both amplitude and frequency and avoids the loss of information when these are processed together.

4. *Bispectral analysis (BIS):* A combination of several signal processing parameters including power spectral, time domain variables and a bispectrum (measuring the correlation of phase between different frequency components of the EEG after fast Fourier transformation). These are combined and correlated with clinical behaviour and function under anaesthesia to provide a linear transition across EEG states from awake to an isoelectric EEG using a real number – the Bispectral index. This ranges from 100 to 0 (Table 58.1). BIS has been derived for use with normal physiology under anaesthesia and is not valid with the injured brain.

CLINICAL APPLICATIONS

The commonest application of EEG is in the investigation and management of epilepsy. Although up to 50% of patients with epilepsy may have a normal EEG; the EEG can help confirm the diagnosis, classify the seizure disorder and identify a focal or lateralised epileptogenic source.

EEG AND PREOPERATIVE CARE

Routine EEG identifying the epileptogenic source is often supplemented by 24-hour video-telemetry, which allows simultaneous video and electrical recording of seizures.

ANAESTHETICS EFFECTS ON THE EEG

Inhalational and i.v. anaesthetic agents produce characteristic dose-dependent changes in the EEG. Barbiturates initially produce β activity associated with loss of the normal α rhythm and an increasing amount of θ and δ activity as the depth of anaesthesia increases. Eventually the bursts of activity become interspersed with periods of low voltage on the EEG – burst suppression (Fig. 58.4). The burst suppression ratio (BSR) is a time domain EEG parameter developed to quantitate this phenomenon and is calculated by dividing the time in a suppressed state (i.e. periods

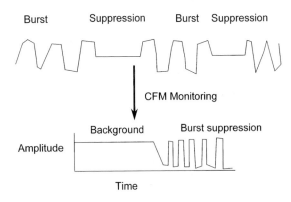

Figure 58.4 Burst suppression, this characteristic pattern consists of bursts of EEG activity which alternate with periods when the EEG is virtually isoelectric. This is also associated with a characteristic pattern on CFM monitoring

within an epoch of ≥ 0.5 seconds during which EEG voltage is ≤ 0.5 µV) by the epoch length.

Other i.v. induction agents with the exception of ketamine, produce a similar pattern with loss of α and varying degrees of β, θ or δ activity. Ketamine activates the EEG at low doses and synchronisation (lower frequency and higher amplitude) at higher doses. Opioids produce an excess of δ and θ activity at high concentrations. Norpethidine (a metabolite of pethidine) is proconvulsant after accumulation.

All inhalational agents activate the EEG at very low concentrations with α activity recorded over the entire cortex, especially the frontal leads. Higher concentrations synchronise the EEG with lower frequencies predominating until burst suppression is reached, followed by an isoelectric EEG when there is maximally suppressed cortical electrical activity. The concentration required to do this varies between agents. This occurs at around 2 MAC for isoflurane, sevoflurane and desflurane, and ≥ 4 MAC for halothane. Enflurane produces seizures above 1.5 MAC dependent on pCO_2 levels (see Chapter 9). N_2O produces a decrease in α amplitude and frontal high frequency activity.

INTRAOPERATIVE EEG MONITORING

Continuous EEG monitoring (normally facilitated by some form of EEG processing such as CFAM) is useful in the following circumstances:

1. *CEA:* EEG patterns correlate with CBF and aid the decision to shunt during cross-clamping. Hypoxaemia produces an acute increase in amplitude of the EEG initially followed by a reduction in amplitude and the appearance of slow waves but may be masked by deep anaesthesia. Persistent EEG changes may predict neurological deficit.
2. *Cardiac surgery:* EEG may be used to detect cerebral ischaemia during extra-corporeal circulation or monitor barbiturates given to provide neuroprotection (see Chapter 40).
3. *Other surgery:* Sphenoidal or foramen ovale electrodes and electrocorticography (direct recording from the cortical surface during surgery) are also useful for epilepsy surgery and evaluation of effects of temporary occlusion of blood flow.
4. *Assessing depth of anaesthesia?* Almost all anaesthetic agents produce a discernible evolution of the EEG as depth of anaesthesia increases. However, the pattern of evolution of the EEG with increasing anaesthetic depth shows a great deal of variation between individual patients and this is not used clinically. BIS correlates with hypnotic endpoints

but is not a depth of anaesthesia monitor or a predictor of movement under anaesthesia. The advantages of BIS may include a reduction in the amount of anaesthetic agent used intraoperatively, a faster wake–up and extubation with more alert and oriented patients in PACU.

EEG IN THE ICU

EEG can be easily performed during intensive care without moving the patient. It is particularly useful in the following circumstances:

1. *Seizure management:* To confirm the diagnosis and detecting subclinical seizures.
2. Diagnosis of certain neurological disorders (Table 58.2).

Table 58.2 Neurological conditions with specific EEG changes

Diagnosis	EEG feature
Creutzfeldt-Jakob disease	Periodic sharp wave complexes
Herpes Simplex encephalitis	Temporal periodic lateralized epileptiform discharges
Subacute sclerosing panencephalitis	Paroxysmal bursts of 2–3 Hz

3. *Outcome prediction:* Certain EEG features are associated with a poor outcome and in some cases may be useful in predicting eventual survival. Various grading systems have been developed based on the presence or absence of these features (Table 58.3). Grades I and II are associated with a good outcome, grade III an intermediate prognosis, grades IV and V are associated with a very poor outcome.

Table 58.3 Grading system for outcome prediction by EEG

Grade I	Dominant α, reactive
Grade II	Dominant θ-δ, reactive
Grade III	Dominant δ-θ, no α
Grade IV	Burst Suppression Low voltage δ, unreactive, periodic general phenomena
Grade V	Very low voltage EEG Isoelectric EEG

4. *Focal neurological disease* detection: This is especially helpful in sedated patients who cannot be examined fully and in patients too unwell to undergo neuroradiological imaging.

5. *Monitoring metabolic suppression:* burst suppression or isoelectricity indicating maximally depressed cortical electrical activity is a useful endpoint following barbiturates given to provide neuro-protection or for refractory intracranial hypertension. Barbiturates may be protective however, before burst suppression is achieved.

KEY POINTS

- EEG represents spontaneous electrical activity of the cortex as recorded from surface electrodes. The principal application of EEG in routine clinical practice is in the diagnosis and preoperative assessment of patients with epilepsy.

- Several automated EEG processing systems have been developed to facilitate interpretation with continuous monitoring, e.g. power spectral analysis, cerebral function monitoring and BIS.

- Continuous EEG monitoring aids the assessment of cerebral function in the anaesthetised patient.

- EEG can be used to diagnose or assess treatment of seizures, status epilepticus, certain forms of encephalitis and raised ICP in the ICU.

FURTHER READING

Rampil IJ. A primer for EEG signal processing in anesthesia. Anesthesiology 1998; 89: 980–1002

Niedermyer E, Lopes Da Silva F. Electroencephalography, 4th Edn. Baltimore: Williams and Wilkins, 1998

Spencer EM. Monitoring of the central nervous system and the effects of anaesthesia. In: Hutton P, Prys-Roberts C (eds). Monitoring in anaesthesia and intensive care. London: WB Saunders, 1994, pp. 256–283

59

TRANSCRANIAL DOPPLER ULTRASONOGRAPHY

B. Matta

PRINCIPLES OF TCD

TCD is a non-invasive monitor that calculates red cell flow velocity (FV) from the shift in frequency spectra of the Doppler signal. This provides *indirect* information about CBF, which can be used both intraoperatively and in the ICU. Changes in FV correlate closely with changes in CBF provided the angle of insonation (the angle between the axis of the vessel and the ultrasound beam) and the diameter of the vessel insonated remain constant (Table 59.1). During anaesthesia, FV also reflects CBF when changes in arterial carbon dioxide tension and BP are minimal and under steady-state anaesthesia.

FV from a number of cerebral vessels can be measured from different locations on the skull (Fig. 59.1). The transtemporal route through the thin bone above the zygomatic arch provides access to the anterior, middle and posterior cerebral arteries. The transorbital approach allows access to the carotid siphon, and the suboccipital route to the basilar and vertebral arteries. The MCA is most commonly insonated because it is easy to detect and allows easy probe fixation providing a constant insonation angle.

Successful transmission of ultrasound through the skull is dependent on ultrasound energy (a 2 MHz pulsed Doppler instrument is best suited) and skull

Table 59.1 Arterial identification and normal adult flow velocities

Vessel	Window	Transducer orientation	Isonation depth	Mean velocity (cm.sec^{-1})	Flow direction from transducer
M_1CA	Temporal	En face	45–60 mm	40–70	Toward
M_2CA	Temporal	Anteriorly	60–75 mm	40–60	Away
ACA	Temporal	Anteriorly	60–75 mm	40–60	Away
P_1CA	Temporal	Posteriorly	60–75 mm	35–55	Toward
P_2CA	Temporal	Posteriorly	60–65 mm	40	Away
VA	Suboccipital	Superiorly & obliquely	45–75 mm	35–45	Away
BA	Suboccipetal	Superiorly	70–120 mm	32–45	Away
OA	Orbital	Slightly medial	40–50 mm	20	Toward
ICS	Orbital	Slightly medial	55–75	40–50	Bidirectional

M_1CA, M_2CA, segments of middle cerebral artery; ACA, anterior cerebral artery; P_1CA, P_2CA, segments of posterior cerebral artery; VA, vertebral artery; BA, basilar artery; OA, ophthalmic artery, ICS, internal carotid syphon. N.B. flow velocity decreases with age.

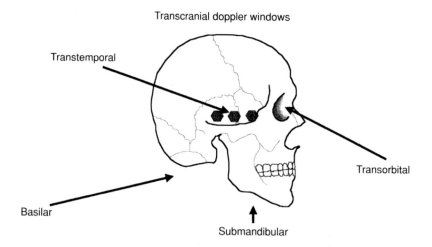

Transcranial doppler windows

Transtemporal

Transorbital

Basilar

Submandibular

Figure 59.1   Optimal locations for insonation (see text)

thickness, which varies with gender, race and age. Approximately 10% of normal subjects can not be assessed through the temporal window. This may approach 20–30% in elderly black females.

FACTORS AFFECTING FV

CBF velocity varies with age, gender and haematocrit.

Age

FV in the MCA is lowest at birth (24 cm/sec), peaks at the age of 4–6 years (100 cm/sec), and thereafter decreases steadily to about 40 cm/sec during the seventh decade of life.

Gender

Hemispheric CBF and FV are 3–5% higher in females, possibly due to a lower haematocrit and slightly higher arterial CO_2 tension.

Haematocrit

FV is also increased in haemodilutional states. When used in isolation, the increased FV observed in these states may be mistaken for vessel narrowing in patients with potential arterial stenotic lesions, such as SAH.

Maximal and mean velocity envelope

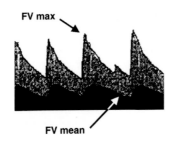

Pulsatility Index = PI

$$PI = \frac{Vs - Vd}{V\ mean}$$

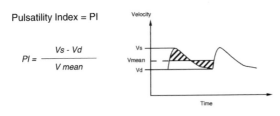

Figure 59.2   Method of determining systolic (V_s), diastolic (V_d) and time averaged mean flow velocity (V_{mean}) from the spectral outline

TCD MEASUREMENTS

A number of measured and derived values are obtained from most commercially available TCD monitors (Fig. 59.2):

FV_{mean}

A weighted mean velocity that takes into consideration the different velocities of the formed elements in the blood vessel insonated. This is the most physiological correlate with actual CBF.

FV_{max}

The maximal peak systolic flow velocity as depicted by the spectral outline. The time-mean FV_{max} is displayed in most commercially available instruments.

Waveform pulsatility describes the shape of the envelope (maximal shift) of the Doppler spectrum from peak systolic flow to end diastolic flow with each cardiac cycle. The FV wave form is determined by the arterial BP waveform, the viscoelastic properties of the cerebral vascular bed and blood rheology. In the absence of vessel stenosis or vasospasm, changes in arterial BP or blood rheology, the pulsatility reflects the distal cerebrovascular resistance. This resistance is usually quantified by the *Pulsatility Index* (PI or Gosling index) = $(FV_{sys} - FV_{dias})/ FV_{mean}$.

Normal PI ranges from 0.6 to 1.1 with no significant side to side or cerebral interarterial differences (Fig. 59.2).

CEREBRAL VASCULAR REACTIVITY

This describes the near linear relationship between arterial CO_2 tension and CBF. In normal individuals, CBF (or FV) changes by approximately 20% for every kPa change in $PaCO_2$.

CEREBRAL AUTOREGULATION

Autoregulation of CBF is a complex process composed of at least two mechanisms operating at different rates; a rapid response sensitive to pressure pulsations (dynamic autoregulation) followed by a slow response to changes in mean pressure (static autoregulation). Both of these processes can be tested using TCD.

The static rate of autoregulation or the index of autoregulation (IOR) is the ratio of percentage change in estimated cerebral vascular resistance (CVRe) to percentage change in mean blood pressure (MBP). An IOR of one implies perfect autoregulation and an IOR of zero complete disruption of autoregulation.

Transient Hyperaemic Response Test THRT

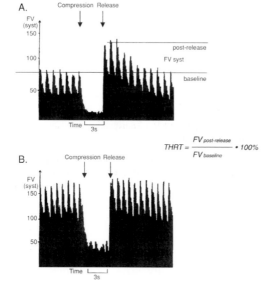

$$THRT = \frac{FV\ post\text{-}release}{FV\ baseline} \cdot 100\%$$

Figure 59.3   Typical middle cerebral artery blood flow velocity response to short compression of the common carotid artery in a healthy volunteer (A), and a patient with impaired autoregulation (B)

Dynamic autoregulation (dRoR) is tested by measuring the recovery in FV after a rapid transient decrease in MBP induced by deflation of large inflated thigh cuffs. The dRoR describes the rate of restoration of FV ($\%.sec^{-1}$) with respect to the drop in BP, in other words the rate of change in CVRe or 'the fast process'. The normal dRoR is $20\%.sec^{-1}$ (i.e. dynamic autoregulation is complete within approximately 5 seconds). Autoregulation may also be tested using the Transient Hyperaemic Response Test (Fig. 59.3).

ESTIMATION OF CPP

FV flow pattern is highly dependent on CPP. The inverse relationship between CPP and PI can be used to non-invasively estimate CPP. Furthermore, when used as a continuous monitor, real time changes in 'true' CPP are easily detected.

TCD IN ANAESTHESIA AND INTENSIVE CARE

CAROTID ARTERY DISEASE

TCD is an important tool in the perioperative care of patients with carotid disease. It allows an assessment of cerebral vascular reserve by examining CO_2 reactivity, detection of pre- and postoperative emboli, monitoring of cerebral perfusion during cross-clamping of the carotid artery, and testing of cerebral autoregulation.

Cerebral ischaemia during clamping of the ICA is considered absent if mean blood flow in the MCA (FV_{mca}) is > 40% of the preclamping value, mild if 16–40%, and severe if 0–15% of the preclamping value.

SAH

TCD is an unreliable measure of CBF in patients with SAH because of vasospasm-associated changes in vessel diameter. However, for a given blood flow, a reduction in vessel diameter is associated with an increase in FV. Therefore, cerebral vasospasm is considered present when $FV_{mca} > 120$ cm.sec^{-1} or the ratio between the FV_{mca} and FV in the internal carotid artery (the Lindegaard ratio) exceeds 3.

TCD can also be used during test occlusion on ICA in patients with giant aneurysms.

CLOSED HI

Following traumatic brain injury, TCD monitoring can be used to observe changes in FV, waveform pulsatility and for testing cerebral vascular reserve. In addition, by continuous recording the FV_{mca}, the autoregulatory 'threshold' or 'break point' (the CPP at which autoregulation fails) can be easily detected. This provides a target CPP value for treatment.

TCD can also be used to diagnose and treat cerebral vasospasm using the same criteria as patients with SAH. Increased FV in combination with high jugular venous bulb saturations ($SjvO_2$) values and FV_{mca}/FV_{ica} ratio < 2 indicates hyperaemia, while high FV within the presence of low or normal $SjvO_2$ values and an FV_{mca}/FV_{ica} ratio >3 suggests cerebral vasospasm.

STROKE

TCD can help identify the source of emboli in acute ischaemic stroke, identify cerebral arterial occlusion, recanalisation and the risk of haemorrhagic transformations of large volume ischaemic lesions. It is possible to identify those patients at risk for further ischaemic episodes by repeated TCD examinations within 6, 24 and 48 hours after admission with acute stroke.

NON-NEUROSURGICAL APPLICATIONS

Because it is non-invasive, TCD has found many applications outside neurosurgery and neurointensive care, mainly in those patients at risk for brain injury secondary to primary pathology outside the CNS, e.g. in pre-eclampsia, cardiopulmonary bypass and hepatobiliary surgery.

KEY POINTS

- Changes in flow velocity using TCD is a non-invasive method of assessing changes in CBF.
- TCD can be used to assess cerebral vascular reactivity, autoregulatory reserve and may be used as an estimation of CPP.
- A high FV indicates vasospasm or hyperaemia. Vasospasm is present if the ratio between the FV_{mca} and the FV in the ICA exceeds 3.

- TCD can be used as an indicator of ischaemia during carotid surgery.
- TCD is a useful tool in patients with SAH, severe HI and stroke.

FURTHER READING

Aaslid R (ed). Transcranial Doppler sonography. New York: Springer-Verlag, 1986

Newell DW, Aaslid R. Transcranial Doppler. New York: Raven Press, 1992

Czosnyka M, Matta BF, Smielewski P, et al. Cerebral perfusion pressure in head-injured patients: a non-invasive assessment using transcranial Doppler ultrasonography. J Neurosurg 1998; 88: 802

Prabhu M, Matta BF. Transcranial Doppler ultrasonography. In: Matta, Menon and Turner (eds) Textbook of neuroanaesthesia and critical care. London: Greenwich Medical Media, 2000

60

APPLICATION OF MULTIMODAL MONITORING

A.K. Gupta

INTRODUCTION

Secondary brain injury may result from raised ICP, inadequate oxygenation or CBF which occur by mechanisms which are complex and multiple. These processes occur frequently and are transient in nature. The purpose of monitoring the brain either in the operating room or ICU is to minimise secondary injury by:

- Detecting harmful pathophysiological events *before* they cause irreversible damage to the brain.
- Diagnosing and effectively treating these harmful pathophysiological processes.
- Providing 'on-line' feedback to guide therapy directed at these processes.

METHODS OF MONITORING

Continuous cerebral monitoring requires a combination of routine systemic methods and specialised techniques specific for the brain:

- *Systemic methods*: These detect systemic changes, which may contribute to secondary brain injury such as hypoxia, hypotension or profound hypocarbia. These methods include measurements of arterial BP, central venous ± pulmonary artery occlusion pressure, arterial blood gases, temperature, pulse oximetry and capnography.
- *Brain-specific methods*: These enable observations to be made of different variables reflecting changes in cerebral haemodynamics, brain oxygenation and metabolism. Current techniques include continuous ICP measurements, TCD, NIRS, jugular venous oxygen saturation ($SjvO_2$), laser Doppler flowmetry and electrophysiology (EEG, CFM). More recently, continuous on-line estimation of brain tissue oxygenation using tissue sensors and brain tissue chemistry using microdialysis have been used. The principles behind these specific methods and their clinical utility are detailed in their individual chapters.

APPLICATION OF MULTIMODAL MONITORING

1. While each of the methods has definite advantages, the drawbacks and limitations of each method are different and do not usually coincide. An example of this is demonstrated in the monitoring of a head-injured patient shown in Figure 60.1. NIRS and $SjvO_2$ are both measures of cerebral oxygenation but the systemic desaturation shown by pulse

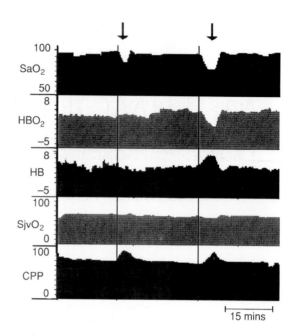

Peripheral desaturation detected by NIRS

Figure 60.1   Changes in oxyhaemoglobin (HbO_2), deoxy-haemoglobin (Hb), $SjvO_2$ CPP and SjO_2 with arterial desaturation (SaO_2). See text for explanation. (Reproduced with permission from M Czosnyka.)

oximetry is not detected by $SjvO_2$, whereas it is reflected by the rise in deoxyhaemoglobin and reciprocal fall in oxyhaemoglobin. A rise in CPP and cerebral blood FV is also seen.

2. Although monitoring of a single modality will yield useful information, it is possible that the observed changes may lead to misinterpretation of events. The addition of other modalities will help to correctly interpret the acquired data and thereby make the right diagnosis. This is demonstrated in Figures 60.2 and 60.3. In Figure 60.2 the rise in ICP is accompanied by a fall in $SjvO_2$, laser Doppler flow (LDF), CPP and FV. This indicates that the rise in ICP was a primary event causing a reduction in CBF. Figure 60.3 shows FV, LDF and total haemoglobin (tHb) rising with an increase in ICP indicating that this was due to cerebral hyperaemia. The ability to differentiate between the two causes of raised ICP has major implications for the direction of treatment.

3. The multimodal monitoring systems allow more reliable decisions to be made intraoperatively. For example brain tissue oxygen sensors in combination with microdialysis has been shown to help determine safe duration of temporary clipping during cerebral aneurysm surgery (see Chapter 56).

Ischaemia resulting from a rise in ICP

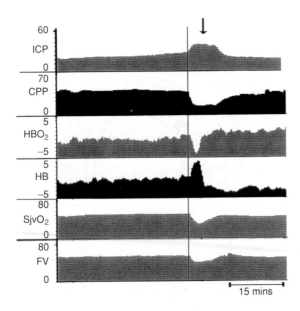

Figure 60.2   Rise in ICP caused primarily by a reduction in CBF. This is demonstrated by a fall in SjvO$_2$, fall in HbO$_2$ and reciprocal rise in deoxygenated Hb measured by NIRS, CPP and FV. (Reproduced with permission from M Czosnyka.)

Hyperaemia induced rise in ICP

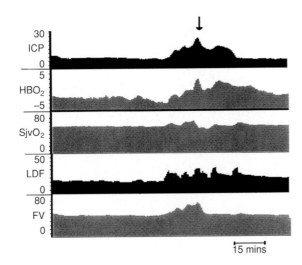

Figure 60.3 Secondary rise in ICP due to cerebral hyper-aemia demonstrated by a rise in FV, LDF, SjvO$_2$ and HbO$_2$. (Reproduced with permission from M Czosnyka.)

4. All monitors are susceptible to artefact which may be difficult to identify in isolation. The multi-modal approach increases the complexity and the potential to generate artefacts in the system. However, since each modality measures independent variables, the artefacts are unlikely to occur at the same time in each modality. Therefore multi-modality monitoring will help differentiate real events from artefact.

5. Although the individual use of TCD, NIRS and cerebral function monitoring have been described for monitoring during CEA, the combined use of these three modalities together with invasive haemodynamic monitoring has enabled thresholds for ischaemia to be defined. This has helped in identifying patients requiring intraoperative shunting.

Multimodal monitoring is expensive. Large volumes of data are generated and computer support for data acquisition and analysis is an essential part of the system. It may be labour intensive for a nurse or technician to ensure that monitors are maintained and remain attached to the patient particularly during long spells of monitoring in ICU.

It is clear that multimodal monitoring enhances the accuracy of interpretation of events and may help in targeting treatment. As experience in these techniques grows, the best combination of modalities which provides sufficient information to help us make early and precise diagnoses and monitor subsequent interventions will become apparent.

KEY POINTS

- Monitoring single variables is useful but has significant limitations.
- Multimodal monitoring gives greater versatility and power of diagnosis.
- Secondary insults of short duration are less likely to be missed.
- General systemic monitoring is part of the multimodal approach.
- Computer support is essential for data acquisition and analysis.

FURTHER READING

Czosnyka M, Kirkpatrick PJ, Pickard JD. Multimodal monitoring and assessment of cerebral haemodynamic reserve after severe head injury. Cerebrovasc Brain Metab Rev 1996; 8: 273–295

Kirkpatrick PJ, Czosnyka M, Pickard JD. Multimodal monitoring in neurointensive care. J Neurol Neurosurg Psychiatry 1996; 60: 131–139

Hutchinson PJ, Al-Rawi P, O'Connel MT, et al. Monitoring of brain metabolism during aneurysm surgery using microdialysis and brain multiparameter sensors. Neurol Res 1999; 21: 352–358

Kirkpatrick PJ, Lam J, Al-Rawi P, Smielewski P, Czosnyka M. Defining thresholds for critical ischemia by using near infrared spectroscopy in the adult brain. J Neurosurg 1998; 89: 389–394

Section 7

MISCELLANEOUS

61

ANAESTHESIA AND MUSCULAR DYSTROPHY

T. Leary

INTRODUCTION

Muscular dystrophies are a group of genetic disorders characterised by progressive weakness and degeneration of muscle, without evidence of denervation.

DUCHENNE MUSCULAR DYSTROPHY (1 IN 3500 MALE BIRTHS)

Symmetrical weakness of the proximal and pelvic muscles is evident from the age of 2–6 years. Contractures and scoliosis develop leaving most wheelchair-bound. Cardiomyopathy, respiratory insufficiency and mental retardation are common. Patients are often referred for scoliosis correction. Death usually occurs at 15–25 years of age due to congestive cardiac failure or pneumonia.

PATHOPHYSIOLOGY

Due to a mutation in the X-chromosome there is an absence of functional dystrophin. The dystrophin-deficient myofibre membrane is unstable and leaky. There is an accumulation of intracellular calcium and cell necrosis. Fat and fibrous tissue replaces the degenerated muscle (pseudohypertrophy). Elevations in serum creatinine kinase are seen from birth (30–300 times normal).

PREOPERATIVE ASSESSMENT

Assessment of cardiorespiratory insufficiency by exercise is difficult. ECG findings include a tall R wave and RSR1 in lead V1, a deep Q wave in lead V3–6, a prolonged PR interval and a sinus tachycardia. Echocardiography may reveal tissue hypertrophy with left ventricular inflow obstruction, posterio-basilar hypokinesis and mitral valve prolapse (25%).

Respiratory capacity falls progressively, and when vital capacity falls below 20 ml/kg, the risk of death is high. Chronic respiratory weakness and a decreased ability to cough result in a loss of pulmonary reserve and accumulation of secretions. Physiotherapy and antibiotics where appropriate are recommended.

INTRAOPERATIVE MANAGEMENT

Suxamethonium should be avoided due to risks of hyperkalaemia and cardiac arrest. Both volatile anaesthetics and suxamethonium have been implicated in rhabdomyolysis and cardiac arrest. Gastrointestinal hypomotility may delay gastric emptying and increase the risk of pulmonary aspiration. Dantrolene should be available and temperature and capnography monitoring are recommended, as there is an increased risk of malignant hyperthermia in these patients.

Intravenous agents, in combination with opioids have been used safely. Non-depolarising agents should be used incrementally with appropriate monitoring, and an awareness of a possible prolonged response associated with skeletal muscle weakness. Regional anaesthesia avoids many of these potential complications and also provides postoperative analgesia facilitating physiotherapy.

POSTOPERATIVE CARE

These patients should be nursed in a high-dependency area. Postoperative insufficiency may be delayed for up to 36 hours. Aggressive attempts should be made to facilitate clearance of secretions including postoperative ventilation until all depressant drugs have been eliminated. Cardiac arrest resistant to resuscitation may still occur.

BECKER MUSCULAR DYSTROPHY (1 IN 33,000 MALE BIRTHS)

This is a X-linked disease associated with abnormal partially functional dystrophin protein. It shows a similar proximal muscle weakness to Duchenne's; however, it is characterised by a later onset (typically aged 16) and slower progression. Cardiac failure due to cardiomyopathy is often the presenting symptom. During anaesthesia, similar precautions as with Duchenne's dystrophy should be adopted.

LANDOUZY–DEJERINE FACIOSCAPULOHUMERAL DYSTROPHY (1 IN 100,000)

This is an autosomal dominant disorder characterised by progressive wasting of facial, pectoral, and shoulder girdle skeletal muscles that begins in adolescence. The course is slow, and lifespan minimally reduced. There is typically no cardiac involvement. Anaesthesia should be directed towards minimising respiratory complications as these patients are at risk of recurrent upper respiratory tract infection.

MYOTONIC MUSCULAR DYSTROPHY (1 IN 10,000)

Myotonia, or the inability to relax skeletal muscle after its stimulation, is the principal manifestation, occurring in the 2nd or 3rd decade of life. However, as the disease progresses, weakness and atrophy become prominent. Treatment is symptomatic with membrane-stabilising agents such as phenytoin or mexiletine. Extramuscular manifestations include cardiac, gastrointestinal and endocrine abnormalities, cataracts, frontal baldness and sleep apnoea. Death from pneumonia or cardiac failure usually occurs by the 6th decade.

PATHOPHYSIOLOGY

There is a dominant inheritance of a mutation in the myotonin-protein kinase gene located on chromosome 19. The result is a defect in sodium and chloride channel function, which produces electrical instability of the muscle membrane. With extended depolarisation, the cellular adenosine triphosphatase system is unable to return calcium to the sarcoplasmic reticulum. Calcium thus remains unsequestered producing sustained muscle contraction. Plasma CK levels are usually normal.

The likely presence of cardiac abnormalities, respiratory muscle weakness, and endocrine abnormalities (diabetes mellitus, thyroid dysfunction and gonadal atrophy) should be expected. Cardiac anomalies include mitral valve prolapse, cardiomyopathy and arrhythmias.

PREOPERATIVE ASSESSMENT

Abnormal responses to anaesthetic drugs should be expected. There may be a need to control cardiac arrhythmias, and temporary pacemakers may be required. Lung function tests and arterial blood gases may reveal the degree of restrictive lung disease. Antacid prophylaxis is recommended as the risk of pulmonary aspiration is increased. The operating theatre should be prewarmed to avoid cold and shivering, both may precipitate myotonia. Adequate monitoring (at least ECG, BP, peripheral nerve stimulator, end-tidal CO_2 and pulse oximetry) should be available at all stages.

INTRAOPERATIVE MANAGEMENT

Induction agents should be used carefully due to enhanced cardiovascular and respiratory depressant effects. Propofol has been implicated in the generation of myotonia. A balanced technique using opioids and inhalation agents is thought to be safe. Ventilation using a cuffed endotracheal tube, should be assisted even for short procedures. Intubation of the trachea may not require neuromuscular blockade,

and should be performed in association with cricoid pressure. Suxamethonium and anticholinesterase drugs are contraindicated as they may produce intense contractures making ventilation and intubation impossible. Short-acting non-depolarising agents, with peripheral nerve stimulator monitoring are recommended. However, they do not consistently prevent or reduce contractures. Contractures may not respond to dantrolene. Regional anaesthesia may prevent exposure to the depressant effects of general anaesthetics; however, it too is no protection from myotonia.

POSTOPERATIVE CARE

There is an increased risk of postoperative complications, including inadequate ventilation, pneumonia and lung abscess formation, pulmonary emboli and cardiac arrythmias. Regional analgesia may avoid the depressant effects of opioids, and allow comfortable physiotherapy. Such patients should be nursed in a high-dependency area.

MYOTONIA CONGENITA AND PARAMYOTONIA CONGENITA

Myotonia congenita is a rare mendelian dominant characteristic manifested in early childhood. It is not strictly a form of dystrophy as there is rarely muscle weakness. The disease, which is limited to skeletal muscle, is one of frequent generalised contractions and muscle hypertrophy. Symptoms respond to quinidine, and there is no reduction in life expectancy.

Paramyotonia is very rare with identical signs and symptoms to myotonia congenita, except that paramyotonia develops only on exposure to cold.

Anaesthetic considerations in patients with these conditions includes troublesome intraoperative contractures, the need to avoid hypothermia and an abnormal response to non-depolarising muscle relaxants.

KEY POINTS

- Muscular dystrophies are characterised by muscle weakness and wasting, without evidence of denervation.
- There is often cardiac and respiratory involvement. Anaesthesia and postoperative care should be aimed at reducing complications within these systems.

- The response to anaesthetic agents may be abnormal.
- Depolarising muscle relaxants should be avoided. Short-acting non-depolarising agents should be used, incrementally, with nerve stimulator monitoring.

FURTHER READING

Aldridge M. Anaesthetic problems in myotonic dystrophy. Br J Anaes 1985; 57: 1119–1130

Smith CL, Bush GH. Anaesthesia and progressive muscular dystrophy. Br J Anaes 1985; 57: 1113–1118

62

MYASTHENIA GRAVIS

S. Senthuran

INTRODUCTION

Myasthenia gravis is an autoimmune disease characterised by weakness of voluntary muscles followed by partial recovery with rest. Sensation and involuntary muscle groups are not involved.

PATHOPHYSIOLOGY

Adult myasthenia gravis is an antibody-mediated autoimmune disease in which IgG autoantibodies are directed against the α subunit of post-junctional acetylcholine (Ach) receptors of the neuromuscular junction. Antibody-negative patients usually have a very mild form of the disease. Thymic hyperplasia is present in 15–20% of patients and thymomas in 10–15% of patients (usually over 30–40 years of age). Removal of Ach receptor (AChr) antibodies by plasma exchange (plasmapheresis) results in rapid improvement of symptoms. Electrophysiological studies show normal frequencies of miniature end plate potentials (suggesting normal pre-synaptic release of acyetylcholine vesicles) but with decreased amplitude, suggesting that the problem is in the post-synaptic response.

CLINICAL PRESENTATION

The disease may present in different age groups with different degrees of severity.

Transient *neonatal myasthenia* occurs in 15–20% of neonates born to mothers with myasthenia gravis. This is most likely to be due to passage of AChR antibody across the placenta but has not been proven. Signs such as difficulty in swallowing, suckling and breathing are usually present at birth but may be delayed for 12–48 hours. The condition tends to resolve within 2–4 weeks with no risk of relapse.

Congenital or infantile myasthenia presents within the first 1 or 2 years of life and is believed to be due to a structural defect in the post-synaptic membrane with a decrease in the AChR insertion sites. It tends to have a non-fluctuating course and is compatible with long survival. As the aetiology is not auto-immune, anticholinesterase therapy is the main treatment.

Juvenile onset myasthenia gravis has an autoimmune basis but without the occurrence of thymomas. It is thus similar to the adult form but is used to refer to the 24% of myasthenia gravis cases that occur before the age of 20. It is slowly progressive with multiple remissions and relapses.

Adult myasthenia has an incidence among adults in the UK of about 1:20,000 and like many autoimmune diseases is commoner amongst women.

The severity of the disease has been classified according to Osserman and Jenkins (1971):

I   Ocular signs and symptoms only.
IIA   Generalised mild muscle weakness.
IIB   Generalised moderate weakness and/or bulbar dysfunction.
III   Acute fulminating presentation and/or respiratory dysfunction.
IV   Late severe generalised myasthenia gravis.

MEDICAL AND SURGICAL TREATMENTS

Cholinesterase inhibitors such as neostigmine and pyridostigmine increase the amount of ACh available at the motor end plate without altering the underlying autoimmune reaction. They are used as first-line treatments and have been found to benefit most patient's symptoms of weakness. Pyridostigmine is more widely used than neostigmine as it has a longer duration of action (5 hours) and causes less parasympathetic effects. Edrophonium is only used in the diagnosis of myasthenia to confirm reversible weakness or when there is doubt as to whether a patient is undermedicated. When edrophonium is given, clinical improvement is seen within 10–60 seconds and lasts from 1–10 minutes. If edrophonium is given to a patient already on anticholinesterases, clinical improvement would confirm undermedication, whereas symptoms such as diarrhoea, hypersalivation, bronchorrhoea, fasiculations and weakness will be indicative of overdosage.

Immunosuppressants such as corticosteroids and azathioprine have greatly improved disease prognosis in the last 30 years. They are indicated for patients whose symptoms are poorly controlled on anticholinesterases. Corticosteroids such as prednisolone or prednisone seem to decrease antibody synthesis and inhibit CD4 T cell proliferation and are effective in up to 80% of patients. They are used in lower doses in ocular myasthenia and in higher doses as first-line treatment for more severe myasthenia.

Azathioprine is effective in 70–90% of patients. It acts more slowly, taking 2–4 months for clinical response to be evident and has fewer adverse effects than steroids. Azathioprine is used when the response to steroids has been unsatisfactory. Azathioprine also decreases anti-AchR antibody titre by inhibition of helper T cell reactivity.

Plasma exchange or plasmaphoresis is used for rapid and temporary improvement in myasthenic emergencies (respiratory/bulbar weakness). Plasmapheresis removes antibodies, cytokines and complement proteins from the circulation. It is effective in 75–80% of patients and improvement lasts from 2 days to 3 weeks. It has been used in preparation of patients for thymectomy or in those unresponsive to other therapies. High-dose immunoglobulin infusion for 5 days is expensive and used in patients with contraindications to plasmapheresis.

Thymectomy is performed in adults with generalised myasthenia and who have either thymic hyperplasia or a thymoma which tends to be locally invasive. Thymectomy is delayed in children until puberty due to possible negative effects on immune system development. Complete removal of thymic tissue is best achieved via a trans-sternal rather than trans-cervical approach. Even small remnants of thymic tissue seem to affect outcome adversely.

ANAESTHETIC MANAGEMENT

Regional anaesthesia using amide local anaesthetics is preferred wherever possible (metabolism of ester local anaesthetics may be impaired in patients on cholinesterase inhibitors). However, general anaesthesia may be performed if some general principles are followed.

The patient should be medically optimised. However, it is controversial whether to continue or stop anticholinesterase therapy preoperatively. Anticholinesterases if continued, may result in potentiation of vagal responses, prolongation of action of suxamethonium and ester local anaesthetics as well as cholinergic crisis. If the patient is on corticosteroids, problems that may arise include: hypertension, hyperglycaemia, poor wound healing, myopathy, cataracts etc. Azathioprine may cause bone marrow depression and liver dysfunction.

Neuromuscular transmission should be monitored so that muscle relaxants drugs can be titrated to maintain 1–2 twitches and thereby avoid overdosage. Infusions of neuromuscular blockers will allow finer control of dosage than boluses which result in greater peaks and troughs. Short-acting neuromuscular blockers such as atracurium or vecuronium are used at one-tenth of the usual doses. The response to suxamethonium is unpredictable. Resistance may arise initially as there are fewer AchR and due to the presence of anti-AchR antibodies. Phase II block may occur at lower doses than usual if the patient is on anticholinesterases.

Facilities for postoperative ventilation should exist if the need arises.

KEY POINTS

- Myasthenia gravis can present at any age and varying degrees of severity, with weakness of voluntary muscles that improves with rest.
- Myasthenic and cholinergic crisis can cause respiratory muscle weakness and distinguishing them can be difficult in practice.
- Medical optimisation prior to surgery may be achieved with anticholinesterases, steroids, azathioprine and plasma exchange. Whether to omit or give anticholinesterases preoperatively is controversial.
- Thymectomy is best performed via a trans-sternal (rather than a trans-cervical approach) and is indicated in adults with generalised weakness and thymomas or thymic hyperplasia.
- Regional anaesthesia is preferred but if general anaesthesia is required, neuromuscular block should be monitored, small doses of short-acting neuromuscular blockers should be used and facilities for postoperative ventilation should be available.
- There may be initial resistance to suxamethonium or a greater incidence of phase II block in patients on anticholinesterases.

FURTHER READING

Baraka A. Anaesthesia and myasthenia gravis. Can J Anaes 1992; 39: 476–486

Evoli A, Batacchi AP, Tonali, P. A practical guide to the recognition and management of myasthenia gravis. Drugs 1996; 52: 662–70

63

AUTONOMIC HYPERREFLEXIA

T. Leary

INTRODUCTION

Autonomic hyperreflexia may be seen in patients with spinal cord injury following resolution of spinal shock and in association with return of the spinal cord reflexes. It is characterised by acute generalised autonomic overactivity, in response to stimuli below the level of the spinal cord lesion.

PATHOPHYSIOLOGY

Autonomic hyperreflexia may occur in up to 85% of patients with spinal cord transection above T6 (the splanchnic outflow). The response is rarely seen in those with transection below T10. The trigger to this instability or mass reflex involving sympathetic and motor hypertonus can be cutaneous, proprioceptive or visceral (such as a distended bladder). Such impulses elicit spinal cord reflexes over the splanchnic outflow tract. In the presence of cord transection, the descending modulation of these responses is lost, producing persistent vasoconstriction and hypertension. Subsequent stimulation of the carotid sinus and aortic arch is manifest as parasympathetic activity. Such activity may produce bradycardia and vasodilatation above the level of the spinal cord lesion.

SIGNS AND SYMPTOMS

Clinical features of autonomic hyperreflexia include vasoconstriction below, and vasodilatation above the level of the spinal cord lesion. Effects of vasodilatation above the level of the spinal lesion may manifest in many ways, nasal congestion for example. Typically, vasodilatation in the intact portion of the body is insufficient to offset the effects of vasoconstriction, as reflected by persistent hypertension. Severe headache, loss of consciousness and seizures may occur. A precipitous rise in BP may lead to cerebral, retinal, or subarachnoid haemorrhage, as well as increased operative blood loss. Bradycardia, ventricular ectopics and heart block may result from increased parasympathetic activity. Left ventricular failure and dysrhythmias may reflect the effect on a heart working against increasing peripheral vascular resistance. These responses may be fatal.

Other problems to consider in patients with spinal cord injury include a tendency to renal failure secondary to recurrent urinary tract infection, respiratory insufficiency, muscle spasm and contractures, poor temperature regulation, gastric haemorrhage and stasis.

TREATMENT

The best management of this condition is prevention. However, should an attack occur, the first stage in treatment involves removal of the stimulus and treating the afferent limb of the response. This may include providing further analgesia, deepening the depth of general anaesthesia or raising the level of regional anaesthesia. Attempts should also be made to reduce the efferent limb of the reflex using ganglion-blocking drugs (trimethaphan), α1 adrenergic receptor antagonists (phentolamine or phenoxybenzamine), or direct-acting vasodilators (nitroprusside). Central-acting antihypertensives such as clonidine are not predictably effective in treating the hypertension associated with autonomic hyperreflexia.

CONDUCT OF ANAESTHESIA

Surgery is a potent stimulus to autonomic hyperreflexia and even patients with no previous history of this response may be at risk during operative procedures. Autonomic hyperreflexia may be seen even in the presence of general or spinal anaesthesia. A 20% perioperative mortality rate for patients with spinal cord transection has been reported. Appropriate vasoconstrictors, vasodilators, as well as drugs that increase or reduce heart rate should be immediately available.

Preoperative intravenous hydration is helpful in preventing hypotension during induction of anaesthesia. Prior to surgery, a thorough assessment of renal, cardiac and respiratory (FEV1:FVC ratio) function should be undertaken to enable planning of both intraoperative and postoperative care.

General Anaesthesia

A smooth induction of anaesthesia is appropriate in these patients in whom sympathetic function is unpredictable. Where muscle relaxation is required to facilitate surgery or intubation of the trachea, non-depolarising muscle relaxants should be used. Between 48 hours and 6 months following the denervation injury, suxamethonium should be avoided. During this time, there may be a fatal hyperkalaemic response reflecting the proliferation of extrajunctional cholinergic receptors.

Local Anaesthesia

Regional techniques may be used alone or as a useful adjunct to a general technique. Both spinal and epidural blockade may be effective at preventing the mass response. However, control of block height may not be easy to attain. Epidural anaesthesia has been used very successfully in the management of labour pain in paraplegics at risk of autonomic hyperreflexia. Epidural pethidine or morphine, in combination with local anaesthetics, have been used as a means of preventing autonomic hyperreflexia during cystoscopy and during labour. Pethidine produces selective blockade of spinal opioid receptors and hence blocks the nociceptive reflexes below the level of cord transection and may prevent autonomic hyperreflexia. Topical anaesthesia is not sufficient for cystoscopy as bladder stretch receptors are not blocked and bladder distension may initiate the hyperreflexic response.

POSTOPERATIVE CARE

Patients with or at risk of autonomic hyperreflexia should be nursed in a high-dependency area. The first signs of the mass response may not be seen until the effects of the anaesthetic start to dissipate.

KEY POINTS

- The response to stimulation in patients with spinal cord transection above T6 may be unmodulated sympathetic and motor activity below the level of the lesion.
- Parasympathetic activity predominates, above the level of the lesion, but may be insufficient to prevent a catastrophic rise in BP.
- Associated disease in other organ systems should be identified.
- Induction of general anaesthesia should be smooth and stimuli kept to a minimum until an adequate depth has been achieved.
- Spinal or epidural analgesia may prevent the mass response, may obviate the need for general anaesthesia and provide postoperative analgesia.
- Attacks should be managed by removal of the stimulus and by using agents to limit the efferent limb of the reflex.

FURTHER READING

Lambert DH, Deane RS, Mazuzan JE. Anaesthesia and the control of blood pressure in patients with spinal cord injury. Anaes Anal 1982; 62: 344–348

Stowe DF, Bernstein JS, Madsen KE, McDonald DJ, Ebert TJ. Autonomic hyperreflexia in spinal cord injured patients during extracorporeal shock wave lithotripsy. Anaes Anal 1989; 68: 788–791

Gronert GA, Theye RA. Pathophysiology of hyperkalaemia induced by suxamethonium. Anaesthesiology 1975; 43: 89–91

Baraka A. Epidural meperidine for control of autonomic hyperreflexia in a paraplegic parturient. Anaesthesiology 1985; 62: 688–690

64

MANAGEMENT OF PATIENTS FOR MULTI-ORGAN DONATION

Q. Milner

INTRODUCTION

The number of heart transplants carried out world-wide is currently static (approximately 3500 per annum) and limited by the availability of organs. Up to 30% of patients on the transplant waiting list will die before surgery. Effective management of the donor not only improves function after transplant but also increases the number of organs suitable for transplantation.

PHYSIOLOGY OF BRAINSTEM DEATH

Asystolic cardiac arrest inevitably follows brainstem death, and is a result of the physiological changes which occur at the time of intracranial hypertension.

CARDIOVASCULAR CHANGES

Progressive rostro-caudal ischaemia in the brainstem initially causes vagally mediated bradycardia, hypotension and a decreased cardiac output. Ischaemia in the Pons adds sympathetic stimulation – the norepinephrine released causing hypertension. This is the classical Cushing response. Destruction of the vagal cardiomotor centre in the medulla oblongata in turn exposes the cardiovascular system to massive unopposed sympathetic stimulation. These changes are known as the 'autonomic storm' and may witness huge rises in plasma catecholamine concentrations. Experimental models have demonstrated increases in plasma epinephrine and norepinephrine of 750 and 400 times normal levels respectively. Profound haemodynamic changes result from the autonomic storm; myocardial work and oxygen consumption exceeds oxygen delivery causing subendocardial ischaemia and myocyte necrosis. Left atrial pressures may briefly exceed pulmonary artery pressures causing distortion of the pulmonary capillary wall integrity, pulmonary oedema and interstitial haemorrhages.

Dramatic though it is, this state of excessive sympathetic activity is short-lived (15 minutes) and is followed by low levels of circulating catecholamines, reduced cardiac output, vasodilatation and hypotension which continues until cardiac standstill.

ENDOCRINE AND THERMO-REGULATORY CHANGES

Destruction of hypothalamic and pituitary function causes hypothermia and neurogenic diabetes insipidus (in response to a deficiency of antidiuretic hormone). Marked decreases in anterior pituitary function occur with low levels of thyroid hormones (in particular tri-iodothyronine T_3) and cortisol. The major metabolic consequence of these changes appears to be at a mitochondrial level with impaired cellular energy production and a shift from aerobic to anaerobic metabolism. Replacement of these hormones has been shown to reverse this switch to anaerobic metabolism and improve haemodynamic function. Some transplant centres now routinely commence infusions of T_3, cortisol, insulin and vasopressin several hours before organ donation.

Physiological effects of brainstem death are summarised in Table 64.1.

MANAGEMENT OF THE DONOR

Prior to the diagnosis of brainstem death care is directed at reducing ICP and preventing secondary brain injury. The declaration of brainstem death is the legal time of death. Once consent for organ transplantation has been obtained a rapid alteration in the emphasis of patient care is required to optimise the function and perfusion of the transplantable organs.

Hypotension is common, resulting from impaired myocardial contractility, hypovolaemia, arrhythmias and the loss of vasomotor tone. Invasive haemodynamic monitoring is recommended to assess organ function and monitor the response to therapy.

Target cardiopulmonary parameters for thoracic organ donation are a mean arterial pressure of 60–70 mmHg and a cardiac index of greater than 2.2 L/min/m^2. High preload should be avoided and pulmonary artery occlusion pressures maintained at less than 14 mmHg. Inotropic support should be weaned

---

Table 64.1 Physiological complications occurring in brain dead patients

- Cardiovascular instability
- Hypovolaemia
- Hypoxaemia
- Metabolic acidosis
- Coagulopathy
- Hypernatraemia
- Hypokalaemia
- Diabetes insipidus
- Hypothermia

to the lowest doses possible once an appropriate volume has been restored with colloid solutions and/or blood. Haemoglobin concentrations are maintained at 10 g/dl and haematocrit at 30%. Normal urinary losses are replaced with 0.18% sodium chloride in 4% dextrose with potassium supplements. Where diabetes insipidus is present replacement of excessive urinary fluid losses is rarely possible and prompt treatment with DDAVP is indicated to prevent hypovolaemia.

Hypoxaemia is a frequent finding in neurological injury, common causes being coincidental thoracic trauma, aspiration pneumonitis, neurogenic pulmonary oedema and pneumonia. It is essential that normal bronchial toilet and physiotherapy routines are continued in the organ donor. Ventilation should be set to achieve normocarbia with tidal volumes of 12–15 ml/kg and positive end expiratory pressure to prevent alveolar collapse. The minimum acceptable PaO_2 for lung transplantation is a $PaO_2 > 30$ kPa when ventilated with a $FiO_2 < 0.6$. However, the lungs should normally be ventilated with the lowest FiO_2 compatible with normal oxygenation. Table 64.2 outlines the minimum cardiopulmonary criteria for organ donation.

Brain dead patients are poikilothermic and active warming is often required to maintain a core temperature above 35°C. The release of fibrinolytic agents and plasminogen activators from the ischaemic brain may cause coagulation disorders and these should be corrected with appropriate clotting factors.

Table 64.2 Minimum cardiopulmonary criteria for organ donation

- MAP > 60–70 mmHg
- CVP / Pulmonary artery occlusion pressure < 12–14 mmHg
- Cardiac index > 2.2 L/m²/min
- Left ventricular stroke work index 15 g/m²
- $PaO_2 > 30$ kPa at $FiO_2 < 0.6$

MANAGEMENT OF THE DONOR OPERATION

The operation to harvest thoracic and abdominal organs is a major surgical procedure lasting 4–5 hours and involving the coordination of several separate surgical teams. Significant blood loss can occur and 4 units of cross-matched blood should be available. The continuation of high quality care is required to optimise the function of transplantable organs. Controversy exists as to whether anaesthesia is required in a patient with no brainstem function; and spinal reflexes may cause hypertension and muscular contractions during surgery. Neuromuscular blocking agents are commonly used. Direct acting vasodilators or a volatile anaesthetic agent may be used to treat hypertension.

The thoracic organs are normally inspected directly after sternotomy to confirm the adequacy of function and full expansion of the lungs, after which the abdominal organs are mobilised. The thoracic organs are removed first, following full heparinisation and cardioplegic cardiac arrest and subsequently the abdominal organs are excised.

KEY POINTS

- Profound haemodynamic changes occur after brainstem death due to a surge of catecholamines.
- Control of body temperature is lost.
- Hormone replacement is usually required.
- Muscle relaxation is required during donation.
- Organ perfusion and oxygenation needs to be optimised prior to donation.

FURTHER READING

Milner QJW, Vuylsteke A, Ismail F, Ismail-Zade I, Latimer RD. ICU resuscitation of the multi-organ donor. Br J Intens Care 1997; 7: 49–54

Power BM, Van Heerden PV. The physiological changes associated with brain death – current concepts and implications for the treatment of the brain dead organ donor. Anaes Intens Care 1995; 23: 26–36

65

BASIC CONCEPTS OF NEUROIMAGING

J.H. Gillard

INTRODUCTION

Imaging for patients requiring neurocritical care who have not had surgery is usually performed in trauma and SAH. The primary objectives of imaging focus on clearing the cervical spine and defining the extent and prognosis of any intracranial injury. This involves the use of plain films and CT. Postoperative imaging is primarily performed to assess haemorrhage, mass effect and cerebral oedema.

SPINAL TRAUMA

There is a high incidence of cervical spine injury associated with cases of multiple trauma. A lateral cervical spine radiograph is invariably obtained in the Accident and Emergency Department on admission. Further views involve an antero-posterior (AP) projection of the whole cervical spine as well as an open mouth AP projection to demonstrate the C1/C2 articulation. Tracing curves connecting the anatomical landmarks outlined in Table 65.1 is a simple and essential part of interpretation (Fig. 65.1). The presence of a step in one of these lines or soft tissue swelling suggests a fracture or dislocation. It is important to ensure that the C7/T1 junction is imaged; a dedicated swimmer's projection or oblique trauma projections are sometimes necessary. CT, with two-dimensional (2D) and three-dimensional (3D) reconstructions can be very helpful in confirming or excluding an underlying fracture provided that it is used in a targeted manner. Figure 65.2 demonstrates a unilateral facet dislocation of C2 on C3 where the inferior facet of C2 has moved anteriorly, becoming perched on the anterior border of the underlying superior facet of C3.

Normal soft tissue accounts for approximately one-third of the width of the vertebral body from C1 to

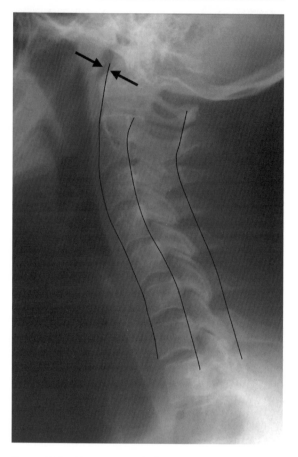

Figure 65.1   Demonstrates the lines connecting the anterior and posterior margins of the vertebral bodies, as well as the bases of the spinous processes. A further smooth curve can be traced between the tips of the spinous processes. The space between the odontoid peg and C1 should measure 3 mm or less in an adult (arrows)

Table 65.1 Assessing the cervical spine radiograph

Lateral projection	Frontal (AP) projection
• Alignment of the anterior margins of vertebral bodies • Alignment of the posterior margins of vertebral bodies • Facet joint alignment • Alignment of the tips of spinous processes • Pre-vertebral soft tissue swelling (does not exclude a significant injury) • C7/T1 included • Vertebral body height equal from C2 to C7 • Intervertebral disk spaces should be equal	• Orientation of the spinous processes • Distance between spinous processes should be equal • Orientation of the facet joints • The lateral margins of C1 should be in alignment with those of C2

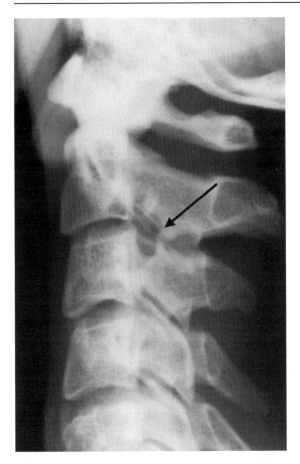

Figure 65.2 Demonstrates facet dislocation with the inferior facet of C2 subluxed and perched on the anterior border of the superior facet of C3 (arrow)

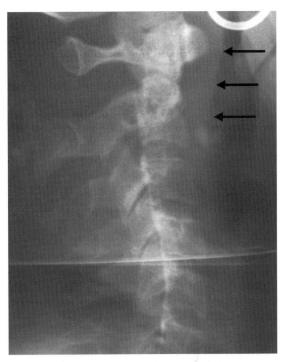

Figure 65.3 This demonstrates soft tissue swelling anterior to C1 and C2 (arrows). There is also slight disruption in the smooth curves of the anterior and posterior vertebral lines. Although these findings are suggestive of an underlying injury, no definite fracture is seen

C4, and up to the whole width of the vertebral body from C5 to C7. Figure 65.3 demonstrates abnormal disruption of the anterior vertebral line as well as soft tissue swelling suggesting an underlying fracture. A subsequent CT reconstructed in 3D clearly shows a fracture through the body of C2 (Fig. 65.4).

In cases of suspected ligamentous injury, flexion and extension radiographs should be considered. Alternatively, MRI has a role in evaluating ligamentous injury. It should be remembered that cervical trauma might also lead to intracranial consequences resulting from dissection of the carotid or vertebral arteries.

INTRACRANIAL APPEARANCES IN TRAUMA

The main aims of CT in head injury are to define the type and site of haemorrhage, to evaluate depressed skull fractures and recognise complications such as cerebral oedema and brain herniation. CT, even with bone window views, is relatively insensitive in demonstrating non-depressed skull fractures. Indications for an urgent CT are described in Table 65.2. Haemorrhage is either parenchymal, e.g. contusions (including contre cous injuries), or extraaxial, either subdural or extradural haematomas.

A classical, biconvex extradural haematoma is shown in Figure 65.5. These are associated with a temporal

Table 65.2 Indications for urgent CT in acute head injury*

- Deteriorating consciousness
- Deteriorating neurological signs
- Confusion or coma
- Tense fontanelle or sutural diastasis
- Open or penetrating injury
- Depressed or compound fracture
- Fracture of the skull base

* In: Making the best use of a department of clinical radiology. Royal College of Radiologists London, 1998.

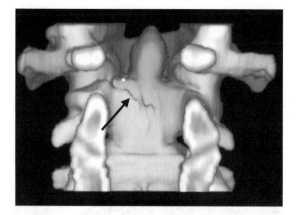

Figure 65.4   A 3D reconstruction of a high resolution CT of C2 clearly demonstrates a fracture through the body of C2 (arrow)

bone fracture in up to 90% of cases (Fig. 65.6) and tend to respect the cranial sutures. It is important for the bone window CT images to be reviewed. Sixty per cent are associated with a tear to the middle meningeal artery, the remaining 40% due to trauma to venous structures. A lucid interval after injury is a frequent occurrence, possibly as a result of slow blood loss or initial hypotension.

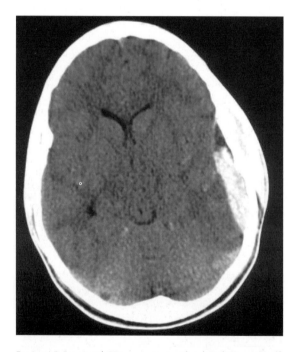

Figure 65.5   Axial CT in a patient with a head injury clearly demonstrating a left temporal extradural collection. There is mass effect, with effacement of the underlying sulci, and left lateral ventricle

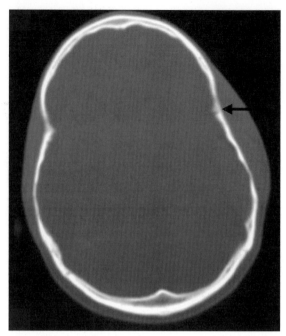

Figure 65.6   Review of the bone windows in the same patient as Figure 65.5, demonstrates a left temporal fracture

Subdural haematomas are associated with significant head injury; up to 30% of patients with severe head injury will have a subdural collection. They are much more common than extradural haematomas, and result from shearing of bridging veins. Collections are concave medially, and do not respect suture lines. Although in the acute stage, blood is dense on CT, untreated they become isodense to normal brain before becoming hypodense in the chronic stage. This can lead to diagnostic confusion. The most common site for subdural collections is over the frontal convexities, but collections can occur in the tentorium, posterior and middle cranial fossae. MRI can be more sensitive in delineating these collections.

Diffuse axonal injury is associated with poor outcome in acute head injury and is associated with shearing of axons and disruption of white matter tracts. Severe cases will be unconscious from the time of injury. There are certain sites that are associated with axonal injury including the body and splenium of the corpus callosum, the brainstem in the region of the superior cerebellar peduncle and the internal capsule. Periventricular injury (Fig. 65.7) may result in intraventricular haemorrhage. There may be parenchymal haematoma or SAH. Severe hyperextension injuries may result in axonal damage to the cerebral peduncles and at the pontomedullary junction. MRI is more sensitive in identifying diffuse axonal injury.

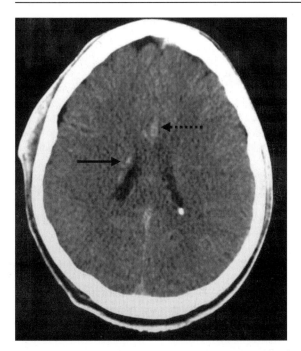

Figure 65.7   A car dragged this 33-year-old patient after a road traffic accident. The CT demonstrates blood products in the corpus callosum (interrupted arrow) and the periventricular white matter (arrow). There is an associated right fronto-temporal soft tissue swelling. Other slices of the CT show subarachnoid and parenchymal haemorrhage, and a small subdural haematoma

SUBARACHNOID HAEMORRHAGE

SAH is mostly due to rupture of an aneurysm (Table 65.3) or arterio-venous malformation. They are less commonly associated with dural malformations, haemorrhagic tumour, trauma or bleeding diatheses. Initial diagnosis is invariably by CT, where hyper-dense blood products are usually readily identifiable (Fig. 65.8), which in expert hands can identify approximately 95% of recent bleeds. Rarely, subacute SAH may appear isodense. In the setting of a good history for SAH, a negative CT without signs of impending brain herniation should lead to lumbar

Table 65.3 Sites of Berry aneurysm in SAH
• Anterior communicating artery • Internal carotid artery (ophthalmic artery) • Posterior communicating artery • Basilar artery • Posterior inferior cerebellar artery

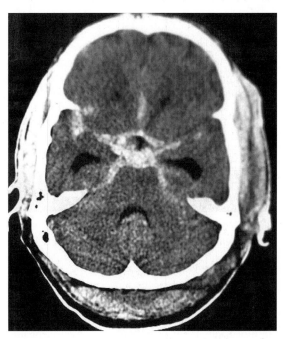

Figure 65.8   This study demonstrates extensive SAH in the supracellar cisterns. The temporal horns are seen, and are dilated, indicating early hydrocephalus

puncture. The extent and location of blood on the CT may be an indicator in identifying the source of haemorrhage. Conventional catheter angiography is usually indicated (Fig. 65.9) and in neuroscience centres is generally associated with low morbidity and mortality. Treatment options include surgical clipping or interventional neuroradiological techniques such as coiling, which is particularly effective in aneurysms of the posterior circulation. Multiple

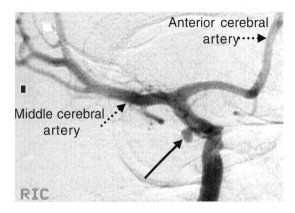

Figure 65.9   The conventional AP angiogram of the patient in Figure 65.8, using selective injection of the right internal carotid artery reveals an aneurysm in the region of the posterior communicating artery (arrow)

aneurysms occur in up to 15–20% of cases. In patients with more than one aneurysm, the presence of an irregular 'nipple' on one of them suggests recent rupture. Not infrequently, no source of haemorrhage is seen on the initial cerebral angiogram, which must include injection into the anterior circulation bilaterally, as well as the posterior circulation. If only one vertebral artery injection is used, this must reflux into the contralateral vertebral artery to identify the origin of the contralateral posterior inferior cerebellar artery. Repeat angiography approximately 5–7 days later may identify an occult aneurysm that may have been tamponaded by local haemorrhage (a yield of approximately 6%). A negative repeat conventional angiogram suggests non-aneurysmal SAH (occurring in up to 15% of cases), which is frequently perimesencephalic. Such haemorrhage is possibly venous in origin and carries a good prognosis.

SAH may be associated with cerebral oedema, raised ICP, parenchymal haemorrhage (due to a jet effect) and intraventricular haemorrhage. Intraventricular haemorrhage frequently leads to hydrocephalus.

Management is centred on preventing rebleeding and vasospasm.

RAISED ICP

The brain is vulnerable to swelling because it lies within a rigid skull. Brain oedema will, therefore, result in raised ICP and risks herniation. Herniation of brain can take a number of forms: tonsillar or cerebellar herniation through the foramen magnum, superior vermian herniation, temporal lobe (uncal) herniation, subfalcine herniation and transtentorial herniation. Mass effect can lead to associated hydrocephalus, e.g. effacement of the 4th ventricle, causing dilatation of the 3rd and lateral ventricles as well as uncal herniation causing contralateral temporal horn dilatation. Raised ICP itself causes effacement of the ventricles and CSF spaces (Figs 65.10 and 65.11). The diagnosis of raised ICP can be difficult in young people as the lateral and 3rd ventricles can be small in normal individuals. A lack of sulcal effacement and the presence of normal CSF cisterns makes raised ICP less likely.

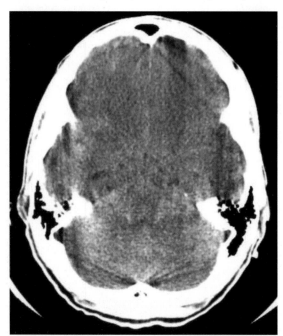 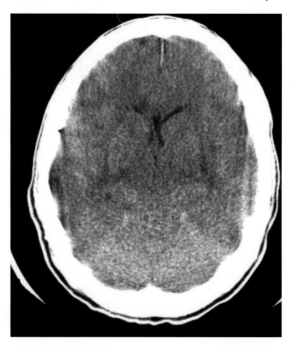

Figures 65.10 & 65.11   These figures demonstrate features of raised intracranial pressure. There is almost complete effacement of the basilar and suprasellar cisterns (Fig. 65.10). The 3rd ventricle is slit like (Fig. 65.11)

66

NEUROANAESTHESIA IN PREGNANCY

P. Popham

INTRODUCTION

Problems involving the brain and spinal cord do occur during pregnancy but fortunately are uncommon. As only case reports or small studies are available to guide management, an understanding of both the physiological effect of pregnancy on cerebral pathology, and the pathophysiological effects of this on maternal and fetal well-being is required. The normal physiological changes of pregnancy influence diagnostic and treatment options and some of these may be unavailable until after delivery of the baby (e.g. stereotactic radioablation using large doses of radiation). Decisions to intervene surgically in non-urgent cases are made depending on maternal health and gestational age. The risk of inducing premature labour as a result of neurosurgery is increased but far less than for abdomino-perineal operations.

PREOPERATIVE MANAGEMENT

To facilitate diagnoses, a high index of suspicion must be maintained at all times, as many symptoms and signs (e.g. headache, nausea, vomiting, tinnitus, dizziness, epigastric pain) are mimicked by the normal physiological changes associated with pregnancy or by conditions that develop during pregnancy (e.g. hypertension, pre-eclampsia and eclampsia).

Exposure of both mother and fetus to ionising radiation in imaging investigations must also be minimised.

Preoperative assessment is viewed in relation to the normal physiological changes of pregnancy. In particular, there is a reduction in functional residual capacity as pregnancy progresses, an increase in maternal oxygen consumption and subsequent predisposition to hypoxaemia, an increase in blood volume, physiological anaemia, tachycardia and thromboembolic tendency and a risk of oesophageal reflux. If consciousness is obtunded, urgent tracheal intubation aids control of ICP and lowers the risk of acid aspiration. Non-urgent intervention should be deferred if possible until at least the second trimester when organogenesis is complete.

INTRAOPERATIVE MANAGEMENT

Fetal monitoring is essential. Intermittent auscultation of the fetal heart can be difficult to perform, particularly if neurosurgical positioning restricts access to the abdomen. The most widely used monitoring technique is continuous cardiotocography (CTG). Ominous signs on CTG are loss of beat-to-beat variability, sustained bradycardia (fewer than 100 beats

per minute), sustained tachycardia (greater than 150 beats per minute) and sudden bradycardia unrelated to a uterine contraction. There must be a medical attendant in theatre who can interpret the changes in fetal heart rate, although if ominous changes do take place there may be little that can be done unless the procedure planned combines obstetrics (caesarean section) and neurosurgery.

Anaesthetic care appropriate for the parturient should be given. This includes routine antacid prophylaxis using preoperative ranitidine combined with a non-particulate antacid such as sodium citrate immediately prior to induction of general anaesthesia. A rapid sequence induction with cricoid pressure is required for all women more than about 16 weeks pregnant. Invasive monitoring may be difficult to site in the parturient due to difficulty in their adopting the necessary position. Aortocaval compression must be minimised during induction by producing left uterine displacement using a wedge under the right buttock or tilting the operating table.

Propofol and thiopentone are safe for induction of anaesthesia. The stressor response to laryngoscopy and intubation may be obtunded with lidocaine, fentanyl or a β-blocker, although the latter may cause fetal bradycardia. Fasciculations following suxamethonium may be attenuated if clinically important, using rocuronium or mivacurium prior to administration.

Excessive hyperventilation should be avoided. A reduction in maternal $PaCO_2$ (< 4.7 kPa) causes a left shift in the O_2-dissociation curve reducing fetal oxygenation. At the same time, uterine vasoconstriction impairs fetal perfusion.

There is no evidence to favour the use of either inhalational or intravenous agents for maintenance of the parturient requiring neurosurgery. Maintenance using a propofol infusion has not been implicated in fetal abnormalities. Maternal BP determines fetal perfusion. If a vasoconstrictor is required, boluses of phenylephrine (20 μg) or ephedrine (3 mg) may be used but with considerable caution if an unclipped cerebral aneurysm is present.

Induced hypotension will adversely affect fetal perfusion and judicious use is required. Labetalol is suitable but may cause fetal bradycardia. The vasodilators (e.g. sodium nitroprusside, hydralazine and nitroglycerin) are generally not advised due to adverse effects on CBV and ICP.

Osmotic diuretics can predispose to ICH and dehydration while loop diuretics are safe if maternal dehydration is avoided. There is often a need for a rapid return of consciousness at the end of neurosurgery carrying the attendant risk of aspiration of stomach contents.

SPECIFIC CONDITIONS

1. *Raised ICP in a parturient in labour or requiring caesarean section:* Analgesia is often difficult as systemic opiates suppress respiration and raise PaCO$_2$. Paracervical or pudendal nerve block may be useful in the second stage of labour but carry the risk of fetal compromise. Uncomplicated epidural blockade is acceptable but dural puncture risks catastrophic cerebellar herniation. Caudal anaesthesia has some theoretical advantages but there is a risk of inadvertent puncture of the fetal cranium and it is not commonly used. Caesarean section is best performed with epidural or general anaesthesia.

2. *Hydrocephalus:* Pregnancy increases blood volume and may worsen pre-existing hydrocephalus. Antibiotic prophylaxis is indicated for delivery. Epidural anaesthesia is acceptable in the absence of documented intracranial hypertension.

3. *Benign intracranial hypertension (pseudo-tumour cerebri):* This may occur in 1:1000 pregnancies and recurs in up to 30% of subsequent pregnancies. A uniform increase in CSF pressure throughout the CNS occurs. The aetiology is unclear and the diagnosis is often one of exclusion. Cerebellar herniation following loss of CSF via lumbar puncture is extremely rare and is not a contraindication to regional analgesia or general anaesthesia.

4. *SAH:* SAH is caused by cerebral aneurysm rupture (75%) or bleeding from an arteriovenous malformation (25%) and it is likely that the chance of bleeding from both causes increases with gestational age. The pressure gradient across the wall of the abnormal vasculature determines the likelihood of further bleeding and the aim of anaesthesia is to minimise changes in this transmural pressure and deleterious effects on fetal perfusion.

5. *ICH:* The overall incidence of ICH in pregnancy is 1–5:10,000. It is normally associated with arterial hypertension and is more common in women with pregnancy-induced hypertension or pre-eclampsia. Management is usually conservative and the prognosis is generally poor if the bleed is large.

6. *Intracranial tumour:* The incidence of neoplasm is the same as the non-pregnant population. Surgical management of slow growing tumours may be deferred until the post-partum period. Some fast growing tumours may be sensitive to radiotherapy but this carries the risk of radiation exposure. There is evidence that some tumours (e.g. meningioma) have surface progesterone receptors and may grow more quickly in pregnancy.

7. *Trauma:* Monitoring of the fetal condition is essential, as premature onset of labour is common.

KEY POINTS

- Neurosurgical procedures in pregnancy are uncommon.
- Detailed knowledge of the physiological changes in pregnancy is required.
- These changes may adversely affect neurological pathology and influence anaesthetic management.

FURTHER READING

Finfer SR. Management of labour and delivery in patients with intracranial neoplasm. Br J Anaes 1991; 67: 784

Hudsmith MJ, Popham PA. The anaesthetic management of intracranial haemorrhage from arteriovenous malformation during pregnancy: 3 cases. Int J Obstet Anaesth 1996; 5(3): 189–193

Johnson MD, Zavisca FG. Intracranial lesions. In: Gambling DR, Douglas MJ (eds) Obstetric anesthesia and uncommon disorders. Philadelphia: WB Saunders, 1998

Rosen MA. Anesthesia for neurosurgery during pregnancy. In: Schnider S, Levinson G (eds) Anesthesia for obstetrics. Baltimore: Williams & Wilkins, 1993, pp. 551–562

67

THROMBOLYSIS IN ACUTE STROKE

A. Coles

INTRODUCTION

In 1996, recombinant tissue plasminogen activator (rtPA) was licensed for use in stroke in the USA following the National Institute of Neurological Disorders and Stroke (NINDS) rtPA Stroke Trial. Subsequent studies of rtPA and other thrombolytics in stroke have yielded less positive results and outcomes from larger studies are awaited. Pilot studies are underway of novel thrombolytics, different routes of access and combination therapies with anti-platelet drugs and neuroprotective agents.

Under current guidelines, thrombolysis is given within 3 hours of stroke onset. This means that most patients will present too late for treatment unless the organisation of pre-hospital care and neuroimaging is greatly accelerated. The cost–benefit ratio of thrombolysis compares poorly with that of simply admitting patients to a dedicated stroke unit. It is estimated that only 10% of strokes will be suitable for thrombolysis and just over 6% of these would be saved from death or dependency. This amounts to only 1.2% of the total who die or become dependent each year after stroke. Treating this 10% with rtPA costs £17,300 to prevent one person from dying or becoming dependent. There would be a 12% absolute increase in the chance of minimum or no disability at 3 months but a tenfold increase in early symptomatic ICH.

If streptokinase were as effective as rtPA, the equivalent cost would be £1500. Streptokinase has been studied in three large trials, which together enrolled over 1000 patients. None showed a significant beneficial effect of treatment and all were stopped because of increased mortality in the treated groups. It is too early to abandon streptokinase though; it may be that the dose used (1.5 million IU, the same as that used for coronary thrombolysis) is excessive or that concomitant aspirin use (which was discontinued in the rtPA studies) prejudiced these studies.

A meta-analysis of thrombolysis trials suggests that long-term death and dependency may be reduced from 63% to 56% if rtPa is given within 6 hours of ischaemic stroke.

The main disadvantage is the time taken to assemble the necessary team to perform an angiogram. At present no evidence exists that the intra-arterial route is better than intravenous thrombolysis.

PRACTICAL GUIDELINES

Protocols for intravenous thrombolysis have been established and it is likely that they will be modified by future studies. Patients should have a clinical syndrome suggestive of a thrombotic stroke. The lacunar syndromes seen in hypertensive patients (i.e. pure sensory or pure motor strokes, clumsy hand-dysarthria syndrome etc.) should be excluded. All patients must have neuroimaging (CT or MRI) to exclude an ICH. Some protocols exclude patients with radiological signs of massive infarction, as these patients may be most liable to develop haemorrhagic transformation.

Within 3 hours of stroke onset, 0.9 mg/kg rtPA (maximum 90 mg) is given intravenously. Ten per cent of the dose is given as a bolus followed by an infusion of the remainder over 60 minutes. Thrombolysis should not be given later than 3 hours, or when the time of stroke onset is uncertain. Streptokinase should not be used outside of clinical trials. Exclusions from thrombolytic therapy are shown in Table 67.1.

Although never proven in clinical studies, it is assumed that an excessively high BP might predispose to bleeding, while excessive lowering of BP may worsen ischaemic symptoms. Pre-treatment systolic blood pressure greater than 185 mmHg or diastolic BP greater than 110 mmHg are often taken as contraindications for thrombolysis. Insertion of central venous access, arterial punctures and nasogastric tubes are restricted during the first 24 hours after thrombolysis.

Aspirin, heparin, warfarin, ticlopidine, or other antithrombotic or antiplatelet aggregating drugs should not be given within 24 hours of treatment. Bleeding after thrombolysis should be treated aggressively with cryoprecipitate or fresh frozen plasma.

Table 67.1 Clinical exclusions from thrombolysis

- Current use of oral anticoagulants
- Use of heparin in the previous 48 hours and a prolonged partial thromboplastin time
- Platelet count less than 100,000
- Another stroke or a serious head injury in the previous 3 months
- Major surgery within the preceding 14 days
- Prior ICH
- Gastrointestinal or urinary bleeding within the preceding 21 days
- Recent myocardial infarction

KEY POINTS

- Intravenous rtPA within 3 hours of ischaemic stroke reduces long-term death and dependency by 12%.
- Risk of immediate death from ICH is increased 3%.
- All patients should have neuroimaging prior to thrombolysis.
- Massive cerebral infarct or uncontrolled hypertension are contra-indications to thrombolysis.
- Both intravenous rtPA and streptokinase may be beneficial up to 6 hours after stroke onset.

FURTHER READING

The National Institute of Neurological Disorders and Stroke rt-PA Stroke Study Group. Tissue plasminogen activator for acute ischaemic stroke. N Engl J Med 1995; 333: 1581–1587

Hankey GJ, Warlow CP. Treatment and secondary prevention of stroke: evidence, costs and effects on individuals and populations. Lancet 1999; 354: 1457–1463

Hacke W, Kaste M, Fieschi C, et al. Intravenous thrombolysis with tissue plasminogen activator for acute hemispheric stroke; the European Cooperative Acute Stroke Trial (ECASS). JAMA 1995; 274: 1017–1025

Hacke W, Kaste M, Fieschi C, et al. Randomised double-blind placebo-controlled trial of thrombolytic therapy with intravenous alteplase in acute ischaemic stroke (ECASS II). Second European-Australasian Acute Stroke Study Investigators. Lancet 1998; 352(9136): 1245–1251

The Multicenter Acute Stroke Trial – Europe Study Group. Thrombolytic therapy with streptokinase in acute ischemic stroke. N Engl J Med 1996; 335: 145–150

Donnan GA, Davis SM, Chambers BR, et al. Streptokinase for acute ischemic stroke with relationship to time of administration: Australian Streptokinase (ASK) Trial Study Group. JAMA 1996; 276: 995–996

Multicentre Acute Stroke Trial-Italy (MAST-I) Group. Randomised controlled trial of streptokinase, aspirin, and combination of both in treatment of acute ischaemic stroke. Lancet 1995; 346: 1509–1514

Wardlaw JM, Yamaguchi T, del Zoppo G. Thrombolytic therapy versus control in acute ischaemic stroke (Cochrane review). In: The Cochrane Library, Oxford: Update Software. Updated quarterly

Index

Note: bold page numbers indicate figures and tables